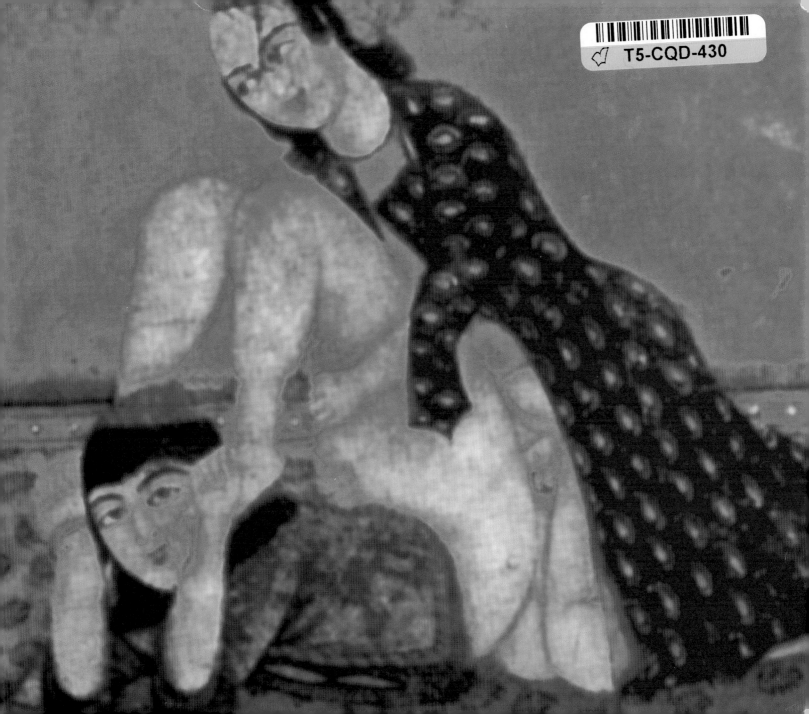

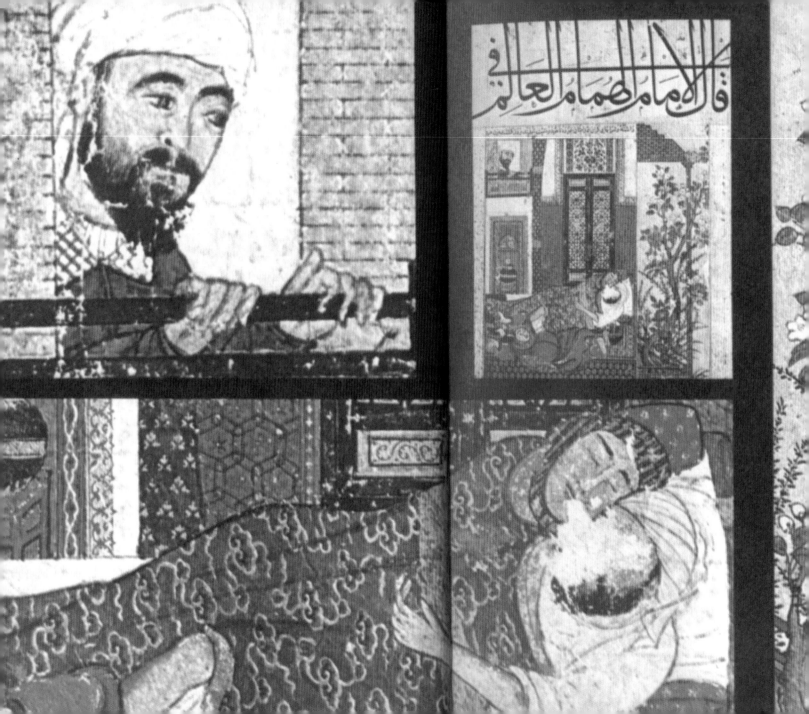

قال الإمام الهمام العالم في

The Perfumed Garden

Erotica behind the harem walls

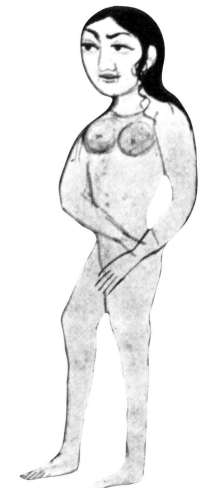

edited by Bret Norton

Astrolog Publishing House

Cover Design: Na'ama Yaffe
Language Consultant: Marion Duman, Carole Koplow
Layout and Graphics: Daniel Akerman
Production Manager: Dan Gold

P.O. Box 1123, Hod Hasharon 45111, Israel
Tel: 972-9-7412044
Fax: 972-9-7442714

© Astrolog Publishing House Ltd. 2004

ISBN 965-494-176-7

Published by Astrolog Publishing House 2004

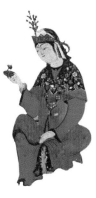

General Remarks about Coition

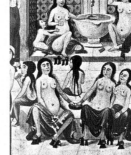

Praise be given to God, who has placed man's greatest pleasure in the natural parts of woman, and has destined the natural parts of man to afford the greatest enjoyment to woman.

He has not endowed the parts of woman with an pleasurable or satisfactory feeling until the same have been penetrated by the instrument of the male; and likewise the sexual organs of man know neither rest nor quietness until they have entered those of the female.

Hence the mutual operation. There takes place between the two actors wrestling, intertwinings, a kind of animated conflict. Owing to the contact of the lower parts of the two bellies, the enjoyment soon comes to pass. The man is at work as with a pestle, while the woman seconds him by lascivious movements; finally comes the ejaculation.

The kiss on the mouth, on the two cheeks, upon the neck, as well as the sucking up of fresh lips, are gifts of God, destined to provoke erection at the favorable moment. God also is it who embellished the chest of the woman with breasts, has furnished her with a double chin, and has given brilliant colors to her cheeks.

He has also gifted her with eyes that inspire love, and with eyelashes like polished blades.

He has furnished her with a rounded belly and a beautiful navel, and with a majestic crupper; and all these wonders are borne up by the thighs. It is between these latter that God has placed the arena of the combat; when the same is provided with ample flesh, it resembles the head of a lion. It is called the vulva. Oh! How many men's deaths lie at her door? Amongst them how many heroes!

God has furnished this object with a mouth, a tongue, two lips; it is like the impression of the hoof of the gazelle in the sands of the desert.

The whole is supported by two marvelous columns, testifying to the might and the wisdom of God; they are not too long nor too short; and they are graced with knees, claves, ankles, and heels, upon which rest precious rings.

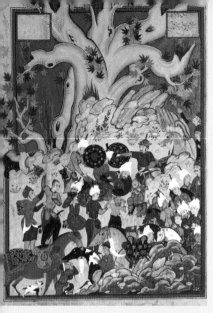

Then the Almighty has plunged woman into a sea of splendors, of voluptuousness, and of delights, and covered her with precious vestments, with brilliant girdles and provoking smiles.

So let us praise and exalt him who has created woman and her beauties, with her appetizing flesh; who has given her hairs, a beautiful figure, a bosom with breasts which are swelling, and amorous ways, which awaken desires.

The Master of the Universe has bestowed upon them the empire of seduction; all men, weak or strong, are subjected to a weakness for the love of woman. Through woman we have society or dispersion, sojourn or emigration.

The state of humility in which are the hearts of those who love and are separated from the object of their love, makes their hearts burn with love's fire; they are oppressed with a feeling of servitude, contempt and misery; they suffer under the vicissitudes of their passion: and all this as a consequence of their burning desire for contact.

I, the servant of God, am thankful to him that no one can help falling in love with beautiful women, and that no one can escape the desire to possess them, neither by change, nor flight, nor separation.

I testify that there is only one God, and that he has no associate. I shall adhere to this precious testimony to the day of the last judgement. I likewise testify as to our lord and master, Mohammed, the servant and ambassador of God, the greatest of the prophets (the benediction and pity of God be with him and with his family and disciples!). I keep prayers and benedictions for the day of retribution, that terrible moment.

The Origin of This Work

I have written this magnificent work after a small book called The Torch of the World, which treats of the mysteries of generation. This latter work came to the knowledge of the Vizir of our mster, Abd-el-Aziz, the ruler of Tunis.

This illustrious Vizir was his poet, his companion, his friend and private secretary. He was good in council, true, sagacious and wise, the best learned man of his time, and well acquainted with all things. He called himself Mohammed ben Ouana ez Zounaoui, and traced his origin from Zounaoua. He had been brought up at Algiers, and in that town our master Abd-el-Aziz el Hafsi had made his acquaintance.

On the day when Algiers was taken, that ruler took flight with him to Tunis (which land may God preserve in his power till the day of resurrection), and named him Grand Vizir.

When the above-mentioned book came into his hands, he sent for me, and invited me pressingly to come and see him. I went forthwith to his house, and he received me most honorably.

Three days after, he came to me and, showing me my book, said, "This is your work." Seeing me blush, he added, "You need not be ashamed; everything you have said in it is true; no one need be shocked at your words. Moreover, you are not the first who has treated of this matter; and I swear by God that it is necessary to know this book. It is only the shameless bore and the enemy of all science who will not read it, or will make fun of it. But there are sundry things which you will have to treat about yet." I asked him what these things were, and he answered, "I wish that you would add to the work a supplement, treating of the remedies of which you have said nothing, and adding all the facts appertaining thereto, omitting nothing. You will describe in the same the motives of the act of generation, as well as the matters that prevent it. You will mention the means for undoing spells (aiguillettes), and to make it resplendent. You will further cite those means which remove the unpleasant smells from the armpits and the natural parts of the women, and those which will contract those parts. You will further speak of pregnancy, so as to make your book perfect and wanting in nothing. And, finally, you will have done your work, if you book satisfy all wishes."

I replied to the Vizir: "Oh, my master, all you have said here is not difficult to do, if it is the pleasure of God on high."

I forthwith went to work with the composition of thi book, imploring the assistance of God (may he pour his blessing on his prophet, and may happiness and pity be with him).

I have called this work, *The Perfumed Garden for the Soul's Recreation* (Er Roud el Aater p'nezeha el Khater). And we pray to God, who directs everything for the best (and there is no onther God than He, and there is nothing good that does not come from Him), to lend us His help, and lead us in good ways; for there is no power nor joy but in the high and mighty God.

I have divided this book into chapters, in order to make it easier reading for the *taleb* (student) who wishes to learn, and to facilitate his search for what he wants. Each chapter relates to a particular subject, be it physical, or anecdotal, or treating of the wiles and deceits of women.

The Perfumed Garden of the Sheikh Nefzaoui

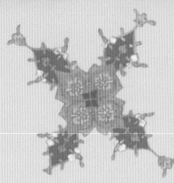

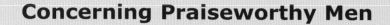

Concerning Praiseworthy Men

Learn, O Vizir (God's blessing be upon you), that there are different sorts of men and women; that among these are those who are worthy of praise, and those who deserve reproach.

When a meritorious man finds himself near to women, his member grows, gets strong, vigorous and hard; he is not quick to discharge, and after the tremling caused by the emission of the sperm, he is soon stiff again.

Such a man is liked and appreciated by women; this is because the woman loves the man only for the sake of coition. His member should, therefore, be of ample dimensions and length. Such a man ought to be broad in the chest, and heavy I the crupper; he should know how to regulate his emission, and be ready as to erection; his member should reach to the end of the canal of the female, and completely fill the same in all its parts. Such a man will be well-beloved by women, for, as the poet says:

> I have seen women trying to find in young men
> The durable qualities which grace the man of full power,
> The beauty, the enjoyment, the reserve, the strength,
> The full-formed member providing a lengthened coition,
> A heavy crupper, a slowly coming emission,
> A lightsome chest, as it were floating upon them;
> The spermal ejaculation slow to arrive, so as
> To furnish forth a long drawn-out enjoyment.
> His member soon to be prone again for erection,
> To ply the plane again and again and again on their vulvas,
> Such is the man whose cult gives pleasure to women,
> And who will ever stand high in their esteem.

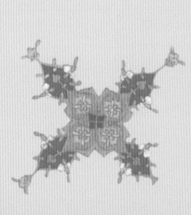

Qualities Which Women Are Looking For in Men

The tale goes, that on a certain day, Abd-el-Melik ben Berouane, went to see Leilla, his mistress, and put various questions to her. Among other things, he asked her what were the qualities which women looked for in men.

Leilla answered him: "oh, my master, they must have cheeks like ours." "And what besides?" said Ben Merouane. She continued: "And hairs like ours; finally they should be like to you, O prince of believers, for, surely, if a man is not strong and rich he will obtain nothing from women.

Various Lengths of the Virile Member

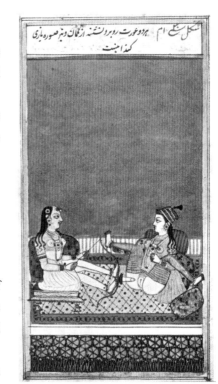

The virile member, to please women, must have at most a length of the breadth of twelve fingers, or three handbreadths, and at least six fingers, or a hand and a half breadth.

There are men with members of twelve fingers, or three handbreadths; others of ten fingers, or two and a half hands. And others measure eight fingers, or two hands. A man whose member is of less dimensions cannot please women.

The Use of Perfumes in Coition.
The History of Mocailama

The use of perfumes, by man as well as by woman, excited to the act of copulation. The woman, inhaling the perfumes employed by the man, becomes intoxicated; and the use of scents has often proved a strong help to man, and assited him in getting possession of a woman.

On this subject it is told of Mocailama, the impostor, the son of Kaiss (whom

God may curse!) that he pretended to have the gift of prophecy, and imitated the Prophet of God (blessings and salutations to him). For which reasons he and a great number of Arabs have incurred the ire of the Almighty.

Mocailama, the son of Kaiss, the imposter, misconstrued likewise the Koran by his lies and impostures; and on the subject of a chapter of the Koran, which the angel Gabriel (hail be to him) had brought to the Prophet (the mercy of God and hail to him), people of bad faith had gone to see Mocailama, who had told them, "To me also has the angel Gabriel brought a similar chapter."

He derided the chapter headed "The Elephant," saying, "In this chapter of the Elephant I see the elephant. What is the elephant: What does it mean? What is this quadruped? It has a tail and a long trunk. Surely it is a creation of our God, the magnificent.

The chapter of the Koran named "the Kouter" was also an object of controversy. He said, "We have given you precious stones for yourself, and preference to any other man, but take care not to be proud of them."

Mocailama thus perverted sundry chapters in the Koran by his lies and his impostures.

He had been at his work when he heard the Prophet (the salutation and mercy of God be with him) spoken of. He heard that after he had placed his venerable hands upon a bald head, the hair had forthwith sprung up again; that when he spat into a pit, the water came in abundantly, and that the dirty water turned at once clean and good for drinking; that when he spat into an eye that was blind or obscure, the sight was at once restored to it, and when he placed his hands upon the head of a child, saying, "Live for a century," the child lived to be a hundred years old.

When the disciples of Mocailama saw these things or heard speak of them, they came to him and said, "Have you no knowledge of Mohammed and his doings?" He replied, "I shall do better than that."

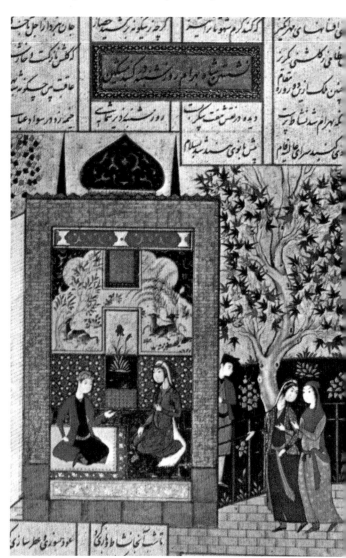

Now, Mocailama was an enemy of God, and when he put his luckless hand on the head of someone who had not much hair, the man was at once quite bald; when he spat into a well with a scanty supply of water, sweet as it was, it was turned dirty by the will of God; if he spat into a suffering eye, that eye lost its sight at once, and whe he laid his hand upon the head of an infant, saying, "Live a hundred years," the infant died within an hour.

Observe, my brethren, what happens to those whose eyes remain closed to the light, and who are deprived of the assistance of the Almighty!

And thus acted that woman of the Beni-Temim form a numerous tribe. She said, "Prophecy cannot belong to two persons. Either he is a prophet, and then I and my disciples will follow his laws, or I am a prophetess, and then he and his disciples will follow my laws."

This happened after the death of the Preophet (the salutation and mercy of God be with him).

Chedja then wrote Mocailama a letter, in which she told him, "It is not proper that two persons should at one and the same time profess prophecy; it is for one only to be a prophet. We will meet, we and our disciples, and examine each other. We shall discuss about that which has come to us fromGod (the Koran), and we will follow the laws of him who shall be acknowledged as the true prophet."

She then closed her letter and gave it to a messenger, saying to him: "Betake yourself, with this missive, to Yamama, and give it to Mocailama ben Kaiss. As for myself, I follow you, with the army."

The next day the prophetess mounted a horse, with her goum, and followed the spoor of her envoy. When the latter arrived at Mocailama's place, he greeted him and gave him the letter.

Mocailama opened and read it, and understood its contents. He was dismayed, and began to advise with the people of his goum, one after another, but he did not see anything in their advice or in their views that could rid him of his embarrassment.

While he was in this perplexity, one of the superior men of his goum came forward and said to him: "Oh, Macailama, calm your soul and cool your eye. I will give you the advice of a father to his son."

Mocailama said to him: "Speak, and may thy words be true."

And the other one said: "Tomorrow morning erect outside the city a tent of colored brocades, provided with silk furniture of all sorts. Fill the tent afterwards with a variety of different perfumes, amber, musk, and all sorts of scents, as rose, orange flowers, jonquils, jasmine, hyacinth, carnation and other plants. This done, have then placed there several gold censers filled with green aloes, ambergris, nedde and so on. Then fix the hangings so that nothing of these perfumes can escape out of the tent. Then, when you find the vapor strong enough to impregnate water, sit down on your throne,

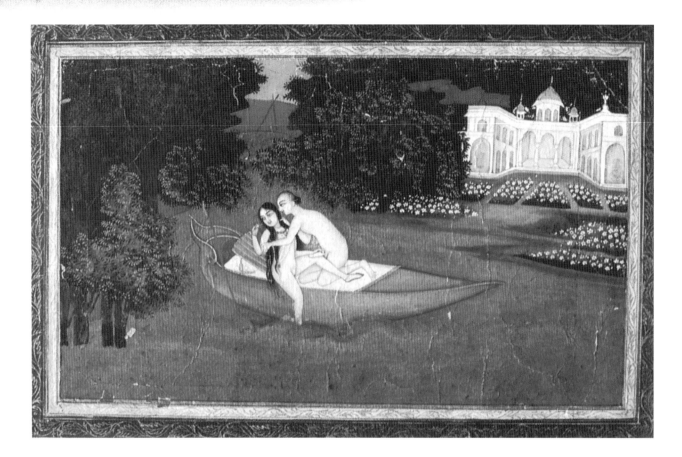

and send for the prophetess to come and see you in the tent, where she sill be alone with you. When you are thus together there, and she inhales the perfumes, she will delight in the same, all her bones will be released in a soft repose, and finally she will be swooning. When you see her thus far gone, ask her to grant you her favors' she will not hesitate to accord them. Having once possessed her, you will be freed of the embarrassment caused to you by her and her goum."

Mocailama exclaimed: "You have spoken well. As God lives, your advice is good and well thought out." And he had everything arranged accordingly.

When he saw that the perfumed vapor was dense enough to impregnate the water, in the tent, he sat down upon his throne and sent for the prophetess. On her arrival, he gave order to admit her into the tent; entered and remained alone with him. He engaged her in conversation.

While Mocailama spoke to her, she lost all her presence of mind, and became embarrassed and confused.

When he saw her in that state, he knew that she desired cohabitation, and he said: "Come, rise and let me have possession of you; this place has been prepared for that purpose. If youlike, you may lie on your back, or you can place yourself on fours, or kneel as in prayer, with your brow touching the ground, and your crupper in the air, forming a tripod. Whichever position you prefer, speak, and you shall be satisfied."

The prophetess answered, "I want it done in all ways. Let the revelation of God descend upon me, O Prophet of the Almighty."

He at once precipitated himself upon her, and enjoyed her as he liked. She tehn said to him, "When I am gone from here, ask my goum to give me to you in marriage."

When she had left the tent and met her disciples, they said to her, "What is the result of the conference, O prophetess of God?" and she replied, "Mocailama has shown me what has been revealed to him, and I found it to be the truth, so obey him."

Then Mocailama asked her in marriage from the goum, which was accorded to him. When the goum asked about the marriage dowry of his future wife, he told them, "I dispense you from saying the prayer aceur" (which is said at three or four o'clock). Ever from that time, the Beni-Temim do not pray at that hour; and when they are asked the reason, they answer, "It is on account of our prophetess; she only knows the way to the truth." And, in fact, they recognized no other prophet.

On this subject, a poet has said:

> For us a female prophet has aris;
> Her laws we follow; for the rest of mankind
> The prophets that appeared were always men.

The death of Mocailama was foretold by the prophecy of Abou Beker (to whom God be good). He was, in fact, killed by Zeid ben Khettab. Other people say it was done by Ouhcha, one of his disciples. God only knows whether it was Ouhcha. He himself says on this point, "I have killed in my ignorance the best of men. Haman ben Abd el Mosaleb, and then I killed the worst of men, Mocailama. I hope that God will pardon one of these actions in consideration of the other."

The meaning of these words, "I have killed the best of men," is that Ouhcha, before having yet known the prophet,

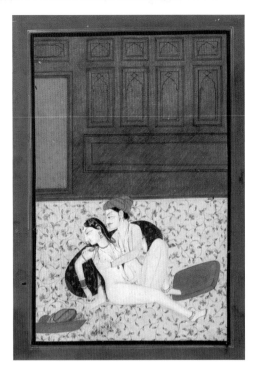

had killed Haman (to whom God be good), and having afterwards embraced Islamism, he killed Mocailama.

As regards Chedja el Temimia, she repented by God's grace, and took to the Islamatic faith; married on of the Prophet's followers (God be good to her husband).

Thus finishes the story.

The man who deserves favors is, in the eyes of women, the one who is anxious to please them. He must be of good presence, excel in beauty to those around him, be of good shape and well-formed proportions; true and sincere in his speech with women; he must likewise be generous and brace, not vainglorious, and pleasant in conversation. A slave to his promise, he must always keep his word, ever speak the truth, and do what he has said.

The man who boasts of his relations with women, of their acquaintance and goodwill to him, is a dastard. He will be spoken of in the next chapter.

There is a story that once there lived a King named Mamoum, who had a court fool of the name of Bahloul, who amused the princes and Vizirs.

On day this buffoon appeared before the King, who was amusing himself. The King bade him to sit down, and then asked him, turning away, "Why hast thou come, O son of a bad woman?"

Bahloul answered, "I have come to see what has come to our Lord, whom may God make victorious."

And what has come to thee?" replied the King, "and how art though getting on with they new and with they old wife?" For Bahloul, not content with one wife, had married a second one.

"I am not happy," he answered, "neither with the old one, nor with the new one; and moreover poverty overpowers me."

The king said, "Can you recite any verses on this subject?"

The buffoon having answered I the affirmative, Mamoum commanded him to recite those he knew, and Bahloul began as follows:

Poverty holds me in chains; misery torments me:
I am being scourged with all misfortunes;
Ill luck has cast me in trouble and peril,
And has drawn upon me the contempt of man.
God does not favor a poverty like mine;
That is opprobrius in every one's eyes.
Misfortune and misery for a long time
Have held me tightly; and no doubt of it
My dwelling house will soon not know me more.

Mamoum said to him, "where are you going to?"

He replied, "To God and his Prophet, O prince of the believers."

"That is well!" said the King; "those who take refuge in God and his Prophet, and then in us, will be made welcome. But can you now tell me some more verses about your two wives, and about what comes to pass with them?"

"Certainly," said Bahloul.

"Then let us hear what you have to say!"

Bahloul then began thus with poetical words:

By resason of my ignorance I have married two wives –
And why do you complain, O husband of two wives?
I said to myself, I shall be like a lamb between them;
I shall take my pleasure upon the bosoms of my two sheep,
And I have become like a ram between two female jackals,
Days follow upon days, and nights upon nights,

And their yoke bears me down during both days and nights.
If I am kind to one, the other gets vexed.
And so I cannot escape from these two furies.
If you want to live well and with a free heart,
And with your hands unclenched, then do not marry.
If you must wed, then marry one wife only:
One alone is enough to satisfy two armies.

When Mamoum heard these words he began to laugh, till he nearly tumbled over. Then, as a proof of his kindness, he gave to Bahloul his golden robe, a most beautiful vestment.

Bahloul went in high spirits towards the dwelling of the Grand Vizir. Just then Hamdonna looked from the height of her palace in that direction, and saw him. She said to her negress, "By the God of the temple of Mecca! There is Bahloul dressed in a fine gold-worked robe! How can I manage to get possession of the same?"

The negress said, "Oh, my mistress, you would not know how to get hold of that robe."

Hamdonna answered, "I have though of a trick whereby to achieve my ends, and I shall get the robe from him." "Bahloul is a sly man," replied the negress. "People think generally that they can make fun of him; but, for God, it is he who really makes fun of them. Give up the idea, mistress mine, and take care that you do not fall into the snare which you intend setting for him."

But Hamdonna said again. "It must be done!" She then sent her negress to Bahloul, to tellhim that he should come to her.

He said, "By the blessing of God, to him who calls you, you shall make answer," and went to Hamdonna.

Hamdonna welcomed him and said: "Oh, Bahloul, I believe you come to hear me sing." He replied: "Most certainly, oh, my mistress! You have a marvelous gift for singing."

"I also think that after having listened to my songs, you will be pleased to take some refreshments."

"Yes," said he.

Then she began to sing admirably, so as to make people who listened die with love.

After Bahloul had heard her sing, refreshments were served; he ate, and he drank. Then she said to him: "I do not

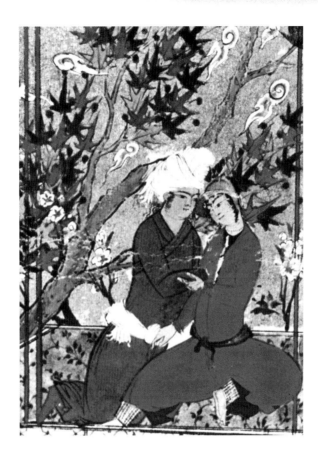

know why, buy I fancy you would gladly take off your robe, to make me a present of it." And Bahloul answered: Oh, my mistress! I have sworn to give it to her to whom I have done as a man does to a woman."

"Do you know what that is, Bahloul?" said she?

"Do I know it?" replied he. "I, who am instructing God's creatures in that science? It is I who make them copulate in love, who initiate them in the delights a female can give, show them how one must caress a woman, and what will excite and satisfy her. Oh, my mistress, who should know the art of coition if it is not I?"

Hamdonna was the daughter of Mamoum, and the wife of the Grand Vizir. She was endowned with the most perfect beauty; of a superb figure and harmonious form. No one in her time surpassed her in grace and perfection. Heroes on seeing her became humble and submissive, and looked down to the ground for fear of temptation, so many charms and perfections had God lavished on her. Those who looked steadily at her were troubled in their mind, and oh! How many heroes imperiled themselves for her sake. For this very reason Bahloul had always avoided meeting her for fear of succumbing to the temptation; and, apprehensive for his peace of mind, had never, until then, been in her presence.

Bahloul began to converse with her. Now he looked at her and anon bent his eyes to the ground, fearful of not being able to command his passion. Hamdonna burnt with desire to have the robe, and he would not give it up without being paid for it.

"What price do you demand," she asked. To which he replied, "Coition, O apple of my eye."

"You know what that is, O Bahloul?" said she.

"By God," he creid; "no man knows women better than I; they are the occupation of my life. No one has studied all their concerns more than I. I know what they are fond of; for learn, oh, lady mine, that men choose different occupations according to their genius and their bent. The one takes, the other gives; this one sells, the other buys. My only thought is of love and of the possesson of beautiful women. I heal those that are lovesick, and carry a solace to their thirsting vaginas."

Hamdonna was surprised at his words and the sweetness of his language. "Could you recite me some verses on this subject?" she asked.

"Certainly," he answered.

"Very well, O Bahlou. Let me hear what you have to say." Bahloul recited as follows:

> Men are divided according to their affairs and doings;
> Some are always in spirits and joyful, others in tears.
> There are those whose life is restless and full of misery,
> While, on the contrary, other are steeped in good fortune,
> Always in luck's happy way, and favored in all things.
> I alone am indifferent to all such matters.
> What care I for Turkomans, Persians, and Arabs?
> My whole ambition is in love and coition with women,

No doubt nor mistake about that!

If my member is without vulva, my state becomes frightful,

My heart then burns with a fire which cannot be quenched.

Look at my member erect! There it is – admire its beauty!

It calms the heat of love and quenches the hottest fires

By its movement in and out between your thighs.

Oh, my hope and my apple, oh, noble and generous lady,

If one time will not suffice to appease thy fire,

I shall do it again, so as to give satisfaction;

No one may reproach thee, for all the world does the same.

But if you choose to deny me, then send me away!

Chase me away from thy presence without any fear or remorse!

Yet, bethink thee, and speak and augment not my trouble,

But, in the name of God, forgive me and do not reproach me.

While I am here let thy words be kind and forgiving.

Let them not fall upon like sword-blades, keen and cuffing!

Let me come to you and do not repel me.

Let me come to you like one that brings drink to the thirsty;

Hasten and let my hungry eyes look at thy bosom.

Do not withhold from me my love's joys, and do not be bashful.

Give yourself up to me – I shall never ause you trouble,

Even were you to fill me with sickness from head to foot.

I shall always remain as I am, and you as you are,

Knowing that I am the servant, and you are the mistress ever.
Then shall our love be veiled? It shall be hidden for all time,
For I keep it a secret and I shall be mut and mizzled.
It is by God's will that everything happens,
And he has filled me with love; but today my luck is ill.

While Hamdonna was listening she nearly swooned, and set herself to examine the member of Bahloul, which stood erect like a column between his thighs. Now she said to herself: "I shall give myself up to him," and now, "No I will not." During this uncertainty she felt a yearning for pleasure deep within her parts privy; and Eblis made flow from her natural parts a moisture, the forerunner of pleasure. She then no longer combated her desire to cohabit with him, and reassured herself by the thought: "if this Bahloul, after having had his pleasure with me, should divulge it no one will believe his words."

She requested him to divest himself of his robe and to come into her room, but Bahloul replied: "I shall not undress till I have sated my desire, O apple of my eye."

Then Hamdonna rose, trembling with excitement for what was to follow; she undid her girdle, and left eh room, Bahloul following her and thinking: "Am I really awake or is this a dream?" He walked after her till she had entered her boudoir. Then she threw herself on a couch of silk, which was rounded on the top like a vault, lifted her clothes up over her thighs, trembling all over, and all the beauty which God had given her was in Bahloul's arms.

Bahloul examined the belly of Hamdonna, round like an elegant cupola, his eyes dwelt upon a navel which was like a pearl in a golden cup; and descending lower down there was a beautiful piece of nature's workmanship, and the whiteness and shape of her thighs surprised him.

Then he pressed Hamdonna in a passionate embrace, and soon saw the animation leave her face; she seemed almost unconscious. She had lost her head; and holding Bahloul's member in her hands, excited and fire him more and more.

Bahloul said to her: "Why do I see you so troubled and beside yourself?" And she answered: "Leave me, O son of a debauched woman! By God, I am like a mare in heat, and you continue to excite me still more with your words, and what words! They would set any woman on fire, if she was the purest creature in the world. You will insist in making me succumb by your talk and your verses."

Bahloul answered: "Am I then not like your husband?" "Yes," she said, "but a woman gets heat on account of the man, as a mare on account of the horse, whether the man be the husband or not; with this difference, however, that the mare gets lusty only at certain periods of the year, and only then receives the stallion, while a woman can always be made rampant by words of love. Both these dispositions have met within me, and, as my husband is absent, make haste, for he will soon be back."

Bahloul replied: "Oh, my mistress, my loins hurt me and prevent me mounting upon you. You take the man's position, and then take my robe and let me depart."

Then he laid himself down in the position the woman takes in receiving a man; and his verge was standing up like a column.

Hamdonna threw herself upon Bahloul, took his member between her hands and began to look at it. She was astonished at its size, strength and firmness, and cried: "Here we have the ruin of all women and the cause of many troubles. O Bahloul! I never saw a more beautiful dart than yours!" Still she continued keeping hold of it, and rubbed its head against the lips of her vulva till the latter part seemed to say: "O member, come into me."

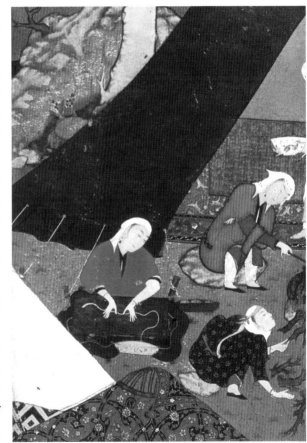

Then Bahloul inserted his member into the vagina of the Sultan's daughter, and she, settling down upon his engine, allowed it to penetrate entirely into her furnace till nothing more could be seen of it, not the slightest trace, and she said: How lascivious has Bod made woman, and how indefatigable after her pleasure." She then gave herself up to an up-and-down dance, moving her bottom like a riddle; to the right and left, and forward and backward; never was there such a dance as this.

The Sultan's daughter continued her ride upon Bahloul's member till the moment of enjoyment arrived, and the attraction of the vulva seemed to pump the member as though by suction: just as an infant sucks the teat of the mother. The acme of enjoyment came to both simultaneously, and each took the pleasure with avidity.

Then Hamdonna seized the member in order to withdraw it, and slowly, slowly she made it come out, saying: "This is the deed of a vigorous man." Then she dried it and her own private parts with a silken kerchief, and rose.

Bahloul also got up and prepared to depart, but she said, "And the robe?"

He answered, "Why, O mistress! You have been riding me, and still want a present?"

"But," said she, "did you not tell me that you could not mount me on account of the pains in your loins?"

"It matters but little," said Bahloul. "The first time it was your turn, the second will be mine, and the price for it will be the robe, and then I will go."

Hamdonna thought to herself, "As he began he may now go on; afterwards he will go away."

So she laid herself down, but Bahloul said, "I shall not lie with you unless you undress entirely."

Then she undressed until she was quite naked, and Bahloul fell into an ecstasy on seeing the beauty and perfection of her form. He looked at her magnificent thighs and rebounding navel, at her belly vaulted like an arch, her plump breasts standing out like hyacinths. Her neck was like a gazelle's, the opening of her mouth like a ring, her lips fresh and red like a gory sabre. Her teeth might have been taken for pearls and her cheeks for roses. Her eyes were black and well slit, and her eyebrows of ebony resembled the rounded flourish of the noun traced by the hand of a skilful writer. Her forehead was like the full moon in the night.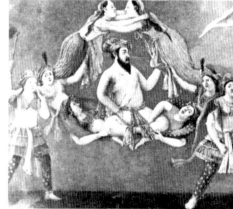

Bahloul began to embrace her, to suck her lips and to kiss her bosom; he drew her fresh saliva and bit her thighs. So he went on till she was ready to swoon, and could scarcely stammer, and her eyes became veiled. Then he kissed her vulva, and she moved neither hand nor foot. He looked lovingly upon the secret parts of Hamdonna, beautiful enough to attract all eyes with their purple center.

Bahloul cried, "Oh, the temptation of man!" and still he bit her and kissed her till her desire was roused to its full pitch. Her sighs came quicker, and grasping his member with her hand she made it disappear in her vagina.

Then it was he who moved hard, and she who responded hotly, the overwhelming pleasure simultaneously calming their fervor.

Then Bahloul got off her, dried his pestle and her mortar, and prepared to retire. But Hamdonna said, "Where is the robe? You mock me, O Bahloul." He answered, O my mistress, I shall only part with it for a consideration. You have had your dues and I mine. The first time was for you, the second time for me; now the third time shall be for the robe."

This said, he took it off, folded it, and put it in Hamdonna's hands, who, having risen, lay down again on the couch and said, "Do what you like!"

Forthwith Bahloul threw himself upon her, and with one push completely buried his member in her vagina; then he began to work as with a pestle, and she to move her bottom, until both again did flow over at the same time. Then he rose from her side, left his robe, and went.

The negress said to Hamdonna, O my mistress, is it not as I have told you? Bahloul is a bad man, and you could not get the better of him. They consider him as a subject for mockery, but, before God, he is making fun of them. Why would you not believe me?"

Hamdonna turned to her and said, "Do not tire me with your remarks. It came to pass what has to come to pass, and on the opening of each vulva is inscribed the name of the man who is to enter it, right or wrong, for love or for hatred. If Bahloul's name had not been inscribed on my vulva, he would never have got into it, had he offered me the universe with all it contains."

As they were thus talking there came a knock at the door. The negress asked who was there, and in answer the voice of Bahloul said, "It is I." Hamdonna, in doubt as to what the buffoon wanted to do, got frightened. The negress asked Bahloul what he wanted, and received the rply, "Bring me a little water." She went out of the house with a cup full of water. Bahloul drank, and then let the cup slip out of his hands, and it was broken. The negress shut the door upon Bahloul, who sat himself down on the threshold.

The buffoon being thus close to the door, the Vizir, Hamdonna's husband, arrived, who said to him, "Why do I see you here, O Bahloul?" And he answered, "O my lord, I was passing through the street when I was overcome by a great thirst. A negress came and brought me a cup of water. The cup slipped from my hands and got broken. Then our lady Hamdonna took my robe, which the Sultan our Master had given me, as indemnification."

Then said the Vizir, "Let him have his robe." Hamdonna at this moment came out, and her husband asked her whether it was true that she had taken the robe in payment for the cup. Hamdonna then cried, beating her hands together, "What have you done, O Bahloul?" He answered, "I have talked to your husband the language of my folly; talk to him, you, the language of thy wisdom." And she, enraptured with the cunning he had displayed, gave him back his robe, and he departed.

The Perfumed Garden of the Sheikh Nefzaoui

Chapter 2

Concerning Women Who Deserve to Be Praised

Know, O Vizir (and the mercy of God be with you!), that there are women of all sorts; that there are such as are worthy of praise, and such as deserve nothing but contempt.

In order that a woman may be relished by men, she must have a perfect waist, and must be plump and lusty. Her hair will be black, her forehead wide, she will have eyebrows of Ethiopian blackness, large black eyes, with the whites in them very limpid. With cheek of perfect oval, she will have an elegant nose and a graceful mouth; lips and tongue vermilion; her breath will be of pleasant odor, her throat long, her neck strong, her bust and her belly large; her breasts must be full and firm, her belly in good proportion, and her navel well-developed and marked; the lower part of the belly is to be large, the vulva projecting and fleshy, from the point where the hairs grow, to the buttocks, the conduit must be narrow and not moist, soft to the touch, and emitting a strong heat and no bad smell; she must have the thighs and buttocks hard, the hips large and full, a waist of fine shape, hands and feet of striking elegance, plump arms, and well-developed shoulders.

If one looks at a woman with those qualities in front, one is fascinated; if from behind, one dies with pleasure. Looked at sitting, she is a rounded dome; lying, a soft-bed; standing, the staff of a standard. When she is walking, her natural parts appear as set off under her clothing. She speaks and laughs rarely, and never without a reason. She never leaves the house, even to see neighbors of her acquaintance. She has not women friends, gives her confidence to nobody, and her husband is her sole reliance. She takes nothing from anyone, excepting from her husband and her parents. If she sees relatives, she does not meddle with their affairs. She is not treacherous, and has no faults to hide, nor bad reasons to proffer. She does not try to entice people. If her husband shows his intention of performing the conjugal rite, she is agreeable to his desires and occasionally even provokes them. She assists him always in his affairs, and is sparing in complaints and tears' she does not laugh or rejoice when she sees her husband moody or sorrowful, but shares his troubles, and wheedles him into good humor, till he is quite content again. She does not surrender herself to anybody but her husband, even if abstinence would kill her. She hides her secret parts, and does not allow them to be seen; she is always elegantly attired, of the utmost personal propriety, and takes care not to let her husband see what might be repugnant to him. She perfumes herself with scents, uses antimony for her toilets, and cleans her teeth with souak.

Such a woman is cherished by all men.

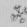

The Story of the Negro Dorérame

The story goes, and God knows its truth, that there was once a powerful King who had a large kingdom, armies and allies. His name was Ali ben Direme.

One night, not being able to sleep at all, he called his Vizir, the Chief of the Police, and the Commander of his Guards. They presented themselves before him without delay, and he ordered them to arm themselves with their swords. They did so at once, and asked him, "What news is there?"

He told them: "Sleep will not come to me; I wish to walk through the town tonight, and I must have you ready at my hand during my round."

"To hear is to obey," they replied.

The King then left, saying: "In the name of God! And may the blessing of the Prophet be with us, and benediction and mercy be with him."

His suite followed, and accompanied him everywhere from street to street.

So they went on, until they heard a noise in one of the streets, and saw a man in the most violent passion stretched on the ground, face downwards, beating his breast with a stone and crying, "Ah there is no longer any justice here below! Is there nobody who will tell the King what is going on in his states?" And he repeated incessantly: "There is no longer any justice! She has disappeared and the whole world is in mourning."

The King said to his attendants, "Bring this man to me quietly, and be careful not to frighten him." They went to him, took him by the hand, and said to him, "Rise and have no fear – no harm will come to you."

To which the man made answer, "You tell me that I shall not come to harm, and have nothing to be afraid of, and still you do not bid me welcome! And you know that the welcome of a believer is a warrant of security and forgiveness. Then, if the believer does not welcome the believer, there is certainly ground for fear." He then got up, and went with them towards the King.

The King stood still, hiding his face with his haik, as also did his attendants. The latter had their swords in their hands, and leant upon them.

When the man had come close to the King, he said, "Greetings be with you, O man!" The King answered, "I return your greetings, O man!" Then the man, "Why say you O man?" The King, "And why did you say 'O man?'" "It is because I do not know your name", "And likewise I do not know yours!"

The King then asked him, "What mean these workds I have heard: "Ah! There is no more justice here below! Nobody tells the King what is going on in his states!" Tell me what has happened to you." "I shall tell it only to that man who can avenge me and free me from oppression and shame, if it so please Almoighty God!"

The King said to him, "May God place me at your disposal for your revenge and deliverance from oppression and shame!"

lWhat I shall now tell you," said the man, "is marvelous and surprising. I loved a woman, who loved me also, and we were united in love. These relations lasted a long while, until an old woman enticed my mistress and took her away to a house of misfortune, shame and debauchery. Then sleep fled from my couch; I have lost all my happiness, and I have fallen into the abyss of misfortune."

The King then said to him, "Which is that house of ill omen, and with whom is the woman?"

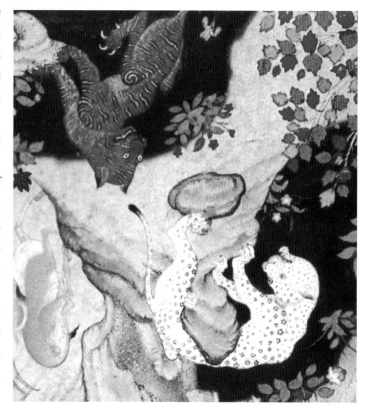

The man replied, "She is with a Negro of the name of Dorérame, who has at his house women beautiful as the moon, the likes of whom the King has not in his palace. He has a mistress who has a profound love for him, is entirely devoted to him, and who sends him all he wants in the way of silver, beverages and clothing."

Then the man stopped speaking. The King was much msurprised at what he had heard, but the Vizir, who had not missed a work of the conversation, had certainly made out, from what the man had said, that the Negro was no other than his own.

The King requested the man to show him the house.

"If I show it to you, what will you do?" asked the man.

"You will see what I shall do," said the King. "You will not be able to do anything," replied the man, for it is a place which must be respected and feared. If you want to enter it by force you will risk death, for its master is redoubtable by means of his strength and courage."

"Show me the place," said the King, "and have no fear." The man answered, "So be it as God will!"

He then rose, and walked before them. They followed him to a wide street, where he stopped in front of a house with lofty doors, the walls being on all sides high and inaccessible.

They examined the walls, looking for a place where they might be scaled, but with no result. To their surprise they found the house to be as close as a breastplate.

The King said to him, Omar, are you determined?"

"Yes, my brother," answered he, "if it so pleases God on high!" And turning to the King he added, "May God assist you tonight!"

Then the King, addressing his attendants, said, "Are you determined? Is there on among you who could scale these walls?

"Impossible!" They all replied.

Then said the King, "I myself will scale this wall, so please God on high! But by means of an expedient for which I require your assistance, and if you lend me the same I shall scale the wall, if it pleases God on high."

They said, "What is there to be done?"

"Tell me," said the King, "who is the strongest among you?" They replied, "The chief of the Police, who is your Chaouch."

The King said, "And who next?"

"The Commander of the Guards."

"And after him, who?" asked the King.

"The Grand Vizir."

Omar listened with astonishment. He knew now that it was the King, and his joy was great.

King said to him, "O Omar, you have found out who we are; but do not betray our disguise, and you will be absolved from blame."

"To hear is to obey," said Omar.

The King then said to the Chaouch, "Rest your hands against the wall so that your back projects."

The Chaouch did so.

Then said the King to the Commander of the Guards, "Mount upon the back of the Chaouch." He did so, and stsood with his feet on the other man's shoulders. Then the King ordered the Vizir to mount, and he got on the shoulders of the Commander of the Guards, and put his hands against the wall.

Then said the King, "O Omar, mount upon the highest place!" And Omar, surprised by this expedient, cried, "May God lend you his help, O our master, and assist you in your just enterprise!" He then got on to the shoulders of the Chaouch, and from there upon that of the Vizir, and, standing upon the shoulders of the latter, he took the same position as the others. There was no only the King left.

Then the King said, "In the name of God! And his blessing be with the prophet, upon whom be the mercy and salutation of God! And, placing his hand upon the back of the Chaouch, he said, "Have a moment's patient; if I succeed you will be compensated!" He then did the same with the others, until he got upon Omar's back, to whom he also said, "O Omar, have a moment's patience with me, and I shall name you my private secretary. And, of all things, do not move!" Then, placing his feet upon Omar's shoulders, the King could with his hands grasp the terrace; and crying, "In the name of God! May he pour his blessings upon the Prophet, on whom be the mercy and salutation of God!" he made a spring, and stood upon the terrace.

Then he said to his attendants, "Descend now from each other's shoulders!"

And they got down one after another, and they could not help admiring the ingenious idea of the King, as well as the strength of the Chaouch who carried four men at once.

The King then began to look for a place for descending, but found no passage. He unrolled his turban, fixed on end with a single knot at the place where he was, and let himself down into the courtyard, which he explored until he found

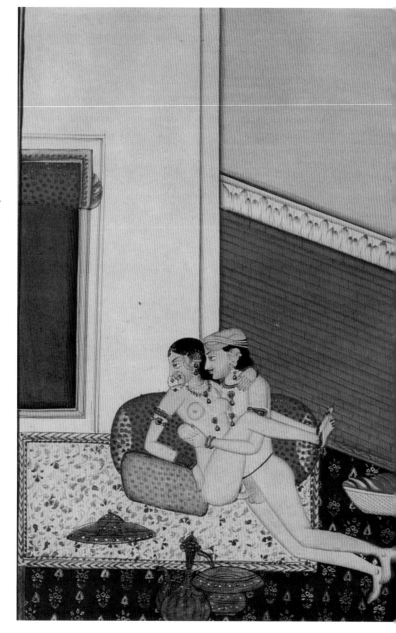

the portal in the middle of the house fastened with an enormous lock. The solidarity of this lock, and the obstacle it created, gave him a disagreeable surprise. He said to himself, "I am now in difficulty, but all comes from God; it was he who gave me the strength and the idea that brought me here; he will also provide the means for me to return to my companions."

He then set himself to examine the place where he found himself, and counted the chambers one after another. He found seventeen chambers or rooms, furnished in different styles, with tapestries and velvet hangings of various colors, from the first to the last.

Examining all around, he saw a place raised by seven stairsteps, from which issued a great noise from voices. He went up to it, saying, "O God! Favor my project, and let me come safe and sound out of here."

He mounted the first step, saying, "In the name of God the compassionate and merciful!" Then he began to look at the steps, which were of variously colored marble – black, red, white, yellow, green and other shades.

Mounting the second step, he said "He whom God helps is invincible!"

On the third step he said, "With the aid of God the victory is near."

And on the fourth, "I have asked victory of God, who is the most puissant auxiliary."

Finally he mounted the fifth, sixth, and seventh steps, invoking the Prophet (with whom be the mercy and salvation of God).

> *Rely not on women;*
> *Trust not to their hearts,*
> *Whose joys and whose sorrows*
> *Are hung to their parts!*
> *Lying love they will swear thee*
> *Whence guile ne'er departs:*
> *Take Yusuf for sample*
> *'Ware sleights [cunning] and 'ware smarts!*
> *Iblis ousted Adam*
> *(See ye not?) thro' their arts.*
>
> The Arabian Nights

He then arrived at the curtain hanging at the entrance; it was of red brocade. From there he examined the room, which was bathed in light, filled with many chandeliers, and candles burning in golden sconces. In the middle of this saloon played a jet of musk-water. A tablecloth extended from end to end, covered with sundry meats and fruits.

The saloon was provided with gilt furniture, the splendors of which dazzled the eye. In fact, everywhere, there were ornaments of all kinds.

On looking closer, the King ascertained that round the tablecloth there were twelve maidens and seven women, all like moons, he was astonished at their beauty and grace. There were likewise with them seven Negroes, and this sight filled him with surprise. His attention was above all attracted by a woman like the full moon, of perfect beauty, with black eyes, oval cheeks, and a lithe and graceful waist; she humbled the hearts of those who became enamored of her.

Stupefied by her beauty, the King was as one stunned. He then said to himself, "How is there any getting out of this place? O my spirit, do not give way to love!"

And continuing his inspection of the room, he perceived in the hands of those who were present, glasses filled with wine. They were drinking and eating, and it was easy to see they were overcome with drink.

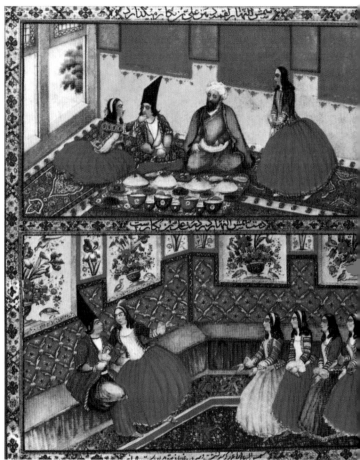

While the King was wondering how to escape his embarrassment, he heard one of the women saying to one of her companions, calling her by name, "Oh, so and so, rise and light a torch, so that we two can go to bed, for sleep is overpowering us. Come, light the torch, and let us retire to the other chamber."

They rose and lifted up the curtain to leave the room. The King hid himself to let them pass; then, perceiving that they had left their chamber to do a thing necessary and obligatory in human kind, he took advantage of their absence, entered their apartment, and hid himself in a cupboard.

While he was thus in hiding the women returned and shut the doors. Their reason was obscured by the fumes of wine; they pulled off all their clothes and began to caress each other mutually.

The King said to himself, "Omar has told me true about his house of misfortune as an abyss of debauchery."

When the women had fallen asleep the King rose, extinguished the light, undressed, and lay down between the two. He had taken care during their conversation to impress their names on his memory. So he was able to say to one of them, "You, so and so, where have you put the door-keys?" speaking very low.

The woman answered, "Go to sleep, you whore, the keys are in their usual place."

The King said to himself, "There is no might and strength but in God the Almighty and Benevolent!" and was much troubled.

And again he asked the woman about the keys, saying, "Daylight is coming. I must open the doors. There is the sun. I am going to open the house."

And she answered, "The keys are in the usual place. Why do you thus bother me? Sleep, I say, till it is day."

And again the King said to himself, "There is no might and strength but in God the Almighty and Benevolent, and surely if it were not for the fear of God I should run my sword through her." Then he began again, "Oh, you, so and so!"

She said, "What do you want?"

" I am uneasy, " said the King, "about the keys; tell me where they are."

And she answered, "You hussy! Does your vulva itch for coition? Cannot you do without for a single night? Look! The Vizir's wife has withstood all the entreaties of the Negro, and repelled him since six month! Go, the keys are in the negro's pocket. Do not say to him, "Give me the keys;" but say, "Give me your member." You know his name is Dorérame."

The King was now silent, for he knew what to do. He waited a short time till the woman was asleep; then he dressed himself in her clothes, and conceled his sword under them; his face he hid under a veil of red silk. Thus dressed he looked like other women. The he opened the door, stole softly out, and placed himself behind the curtains of the saloon entrance. He saw only some people sitting there; the remainder were asleep.

The King made the following silent prayer, "O my soul, let me follow the right way, and let all those people among whom I find myself be stunned swith drunkenness, so that they cannot know the King from his subjects, and God give me strength."

He then entered the saloon saying: "In the name of God!" and he tottered towards the bed of the Negro as if drunk. The Negroes and the women took him to be the woman whose attire he had taken.

Dorérame had a great desire to have his pleasure with that woman, and when he saw her sit down by the bed he thought that she had broken her sleep to come to him, perhaps for love games. So he said, "Oh, you, so and so, undress and get into my bed, I shall soon be back."

The King said to himself, "There is no might and strength but in the High God, the Benevolent!" Then he searched for the keys in the clothes and pockets of the Negro, but found nothing. He said, "God's will be done!" Then raising his eyes, he saw a high window; he reached up with his arm, and found gold-embroidered garments there; he slipped his

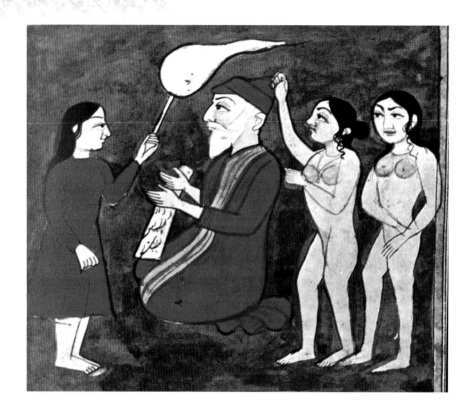

hands into the pockets, and, oh, surprise! He found the keys. He examined them and counted seven, corresponding to the number of the doors of the house, and in his joy, he exclaimed, "God, be praised and glorified!" Then he said, "I can only get out of here by a ruse." Then feigning sickness, and appearing as if he wanted to vomit violently, he held his hand before his mouth, and hurried to the center of the courtyard. The Negro said to him, "God bless you! Oh, so and so! Any other woman would have been sick into the bed!"

The King then went to the inner door of the house, and opened it; he closed it behind him, and so from one door to the other, till he came to the seventh, which opened upon the street. Here he found his companions again, who had been in great anxiety, and who asked him what he had seen.

Then said the King; "This is not the time to answer. Let us go into this house with the blessing of God and with his help."

They resolved to be upon their guard, there being in the house seven Negroes, twelve maidens and seven women, beautiful as moons.

The Vizir asked the King, "What garments are these?" And the King answered, "Be silent' without them I should never have got the keys."

He then went to the chamber where the two women were, with whom he had been lying, took off the clothes in which he was dressed, and resumed his own, taking good care of his sword. Repairing to the saloon, where the Negroes and the women were, he and his companions ranged themselves behind the door curtain.

After having looked into the saloon, they said, "Among all these women there is none more beautiful than the one seated on the elevated cushion!" The King said, "I reserve her for myself, if she does not belong to someone else."

While they were examining the interior of the saloon, Dorérame descended from the bed, and after him one of those beautiful women. Then another Negro got on the bed with another woman, and so on till the seventh. They rode them in this way, one after the other, excepting the beautiful woman mentioned above, and the maidens. Each of these women appeared to mount upon the bed with marked reluctance, and descended, after the coition was finished, with her head bent down.

The Negroes, however, were lusting after, and pressing on after the other, the beautiful woman. But she spurned them all, saying, "I shall never consent to it, and as to these virgins, I take them also under my protection."

Dorérame then rose and went up to her, holding in his hands his member in full erection, stiff as a pillar. He hit her with it on the face and head, saying, "Six times this night I have pressed you to cede to my desires, and you always refuse; but now I must have you, even this night."

When the woman saw the stubbornness of the negro and the state of drunkenness he was in, she tried to soften him by promises. "Sit down here by me," she said, "and tonight thy desires shall be contented."

The Negro sat down near her with his member still erect as a column. The King could scarcely master his surprise.

Then the woman began to sing the following verses, intoning them from the bottom of her heart:

I prefer a young man for coition, and him only;
He is full of courage – he is my sole ambition,
His member is strong to deflower the virgin,
And richly proportioned in all it dimensions;

It has a head like to a brazier.

Enormous, and none like it in creation;

Strong it is and hard, with the head rounded off.

It is always ready for action and does not die down;

It never sleeps, owing to the violence of its love.

It sighs to enter my vulva, and sheds tears on my belly;

It asks not for help, not being in want of any;

It has no need of an ally, and stands alone the greatest fatigues,

And nobody can be sure of what will result from its efforts.

Full of vigor and life, it bores into my vagina,

And it works about there in action constant and splendid.

First from the front to the back, and then from the right to the left;

Now it is crammed hard in my vigorous pressure,

Now it rubs its head on the orifice of my vagina.

And he strokes my back, my stomach, my sides,

Kisses my cheeks, and anon begins to suck at my lips.

He embraces me close, and makes me roll on the bed,

And between his arms I am like a corpse without life.

Every part of my body receives in turn his love-bites,

And he covers me with kisses of fire;

When he sees me in heat he quickly comes to me,

Then he opens my thighs and kisses my belly,

And puts his tool in my hand to make it knowck at my door.

Soon he is in the cave, and I feel pleasure approaching.

He shakes me and trills me, and hotly we both are working,

And he says, "Receive my seed!" and I answer, "Oh give it beloved one!

It shall be welcome to me, you light of my eyes!

Oh, you man of all men, who fillest me with pleasure.

Oh, you soul of my soul, go on with fresh vigor,

For you must not yet withdraw it from me; leave it there,

And this day will then be free of all sorrow."

He had sworn to God to have me for seventy nights,

And what he wished for he did, in the way of kisses and embraces, during all those nights.

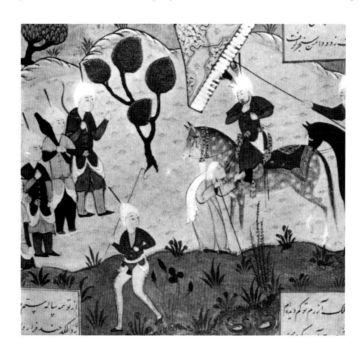

When she had finished, the King, in great surprise, said "How lascivious has God made this woman." And turning to his companions, "There is no doubt that this woman has no husband, and has not been debauched, for, certainly that Negro is in love with her, and she has nevertheless repulsed him."

Omar ben Isad took the word, "This is true, O King! Her husband has been now away for nearly a year, and many men have endeavored to debauch her, but she has resisted."

The King asked, "Who is her husband?" And his companions answered, "She is the wife of the son of your father's Vizir."

The King replied, "You speak true; I have indeed heard it said that the son of my father's Vizir had a wife without fault, endowed with the beauty and perfection and of exquisite shape; not adulterous and innocent of debauchery."

This is the same woman," said they.

The King said, "No matter how, but I must have her," and turning to Omar, eh added, "Where, among these women, is your mistress?"

Omar answered, "I do not see her, O King!" upon which the King said, "Have patience, I will show her to you." Omar was quite surprised to find that the King knew so much. "And this then is the Negro Dorérame?" asked the King. "Yes, and he is a slave of mine," answered the Vizir. Be silent, this is not the timed to speak," said the King.

While this of course was going on, the Negro Dorérame, still desirous of obtaining the favors of that lady, said to her, "I am tired of your lies, O Beder el Bedour" (full moon of the full moons), for so she called herself.

The King said, "He who called her so called her by her true name, for she is the full moon of the full moons, afore God!"

However, the Negro wanted to draw the woman away with him, and hit her in the face.

The King, made with jealousy, and with his heart full of ire, said to Vizir, "Look what your Negro is doing! By God! He shall die the death of a villain, and I shall make an example of him, and a warning to those who would imitate him!"

Ye are the wish, the aim of me
And when, O Love, thy sight I see
The heavenly mansion openeth;
But hell I see when lost thy sight.
From thee comes madness; nor the less
Comes highest joy, comes ecstasy:
Nor in my love for thee I fear
Or shame and blame, or hate and spite.
When Love was throned within my heart
I rent [tore] the veil of modesty;
And stints [stops] not Love to rend that veil
Garring [Causing] disgrace on grace to alight;
The robe of sickness then I donned
But rent to rags was secrecy:
Wherefore my love and longing heart
Proclaim your high supremest might;
The tear-drop railing [flowing] adown my cheek
Telleth my tale of ignomy [disgrace]:
And all the hid was seen by all
And all my riddle ree'd aright.
Heal then my malady, for thou
Art malady and remedy!
But she whose cure is in thy hand
Shall ne'er be free of bane [destruction]
    and blight [damage];

Burn me those eyne [eyes] that radiance rain
Slay me the swords of phantasy;
How many hath the sword of Love
Laid low, their high degree despite?
Yet will I never cease to pine
Nor to oblivion will I flee.
Love is my health, my faith, my joy
Public and private, wrong or right.
O happy eyes that sight thy charms
That gaze upon thee at their gree [pleasure]!
Yea, of my purest wish and will
The slave of Love I'll aye be hight [called].

The Arabian Nights

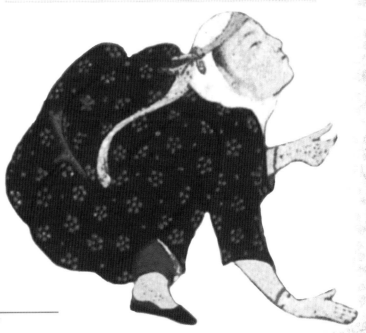

At that moment the King heard the lady say to the Negro, "You are betraying your master the Vizir wth his wife, and now you betray her, in spite of your intimacy with her and the favors she grants to you. And surely she loves you passionately and you are pursing another woman!"

The King said to the Vizir, "Listen, and do not speak a word."

The lady then rose and returned to the place where she had been before, and began to recite:

Oh, men! Listen to what I say on the subject of woman,
Her thirst for coition is written between her eyes.
Do not put trust in her vows, even were she the Sultan's daughter.
Woman's malice is boundless; not even the king of kings
Would suffice to subdue it, whate'er be his might.
Men, take heed and shun the love of woman!
Do not say, "Such a one is my well beloved;"
Do not say, "She is my life's companion."
If I deceive you, then say my words are untruths.
As long as she is with you in bed, you have her love,
But a woman's love is not enduring, believe me.
Lying upon her breast, you are her love-treasure;
While the coition goes on, you have her love, poor fool!
But, anon, she looks upon you as a fiend;
And this is a fact undoubted and certain.
The wife receives the slave in the bed of the master,
And the serving-men allay upon her their lust.

Certain it is, such conduct is not to be praised and honored.

But the virtue of women is frail and changeful,

And the man thus deceived is looked upon with contempt.

Therefore a man with a heart should not put trust in a woman.

At these words the Vizir began to cry, but the King bad him to be quiet. Then the Negro recited the following verses in response to those of the lady:

We Negroes have had our fill of women,

We fear not their tricks, however subtle they be.

Men confide in us with regard to what they cherish.

This is no lie, remember, but is the truth, as you know.

Oh, you women all! For sure you have no patience when the virile member you are wanting,

For in the same resides your life and death;

It is the end and all of your wishes, secret or open.

If you choler and ire are aroused against your husbands,

They appease you simply by introducing their members.

Your religion resudes in your vulva, and the manly member is your soul.

Such you will always find the nature of woman.

With that, the Negro threw himself upon the woman, who pushed him back.

At this moment, the King felt his heart oppressed; he drew his sword, as did his companions, and they entered the room. The Negroes and women saw nothing but brandished swords.

One of the Negroes rose, and rushed upon the King and his companions, but the Chaouch severed with one blow his head from his body. The King cried, "God's blessing upon you! Your arm is not withered and your mother has not borne a weakling. You have struck down your enemies, and paradise shall be your dwelling and place of rest!"

Another Negro got up and aimed a blow at the Chaouch, which broke the sword of the Chaouch in twain. It had been a beautiful weapon, and the Chaouch, on seeing it ruined, broke out into the most violent passion; he seized the Negro by the arm, lifted him up, and threw him against the wall, breaking his bones. Then the King cried, "God is great. He has not dried up your hand. Oh, what a Chaouch! God grant you his blessing."

The Negroes, when they saw this, were cowed and silent, and the King, master now of their lives, said, "The man that lifts his hand only, shall lose his head!" And he commanded that the remaining five Negroes should have their hands tied behind their backs.

This having been done, he turned to Beder el Bedour and asked her, "Whose wife are you, and who is this negro?"

She then told him on that subject what he had heard already from Omar. And the King thanked her, saying "May God give you his blessing." He then asked her, "How long can a woman patiently do without coition?" She seemed amazed, but the King said, "Speak, and do not be abashed."

She then answered, "A well-born lady of high origin can remain for six months without; but a lowly woman of no race nor high blood, who does not respect herself when she can lay her hand upon a man, will have him upon her; his stomach and his member will know her vagina."

Then said the King, pointing to one of the women, "Who is this one?" She answered, "This is the wife of the Cadi." "And this one?" "The wife of the second Vizir." "And this?" "The wife of the Chief of the Muftis." "And that one?" "The Treasurer's" "And those two women that are in the other room?" She answered, "They have received the hospitality of the house, and one of them was brought here yesterday by an old woman; the Negro has so far not got possession of her."

Then said Omar, "This is the one I spoke to you about, O my master."

"And the other woman? To whom does she belong?" said the King.

"She is the wife of the Amine of the Carpenters," answered she.

Then said the King, "And these girls, who are they?"

She answered, "This one is the daughter of the clerk of the treasury; this other one the daughter of the Mohtesib, the third is the daughter of the Bouab, the next one the daughter of the Amine of the Moueddin; that one the daughter of the color-keeper." At the invitation of the King, she passed them thus all in review.

The king then asked for the reason of so many women being brought together there.

Beder el Bedour replied, "O master of ours, the Negro knows no other passions than for coition and good wine. He keeps making love night and day, and his member rests only when he himself is asleep."

The King asked further, "What does he live upon?"

She said, "Upon yolks of eggs friend in fat and swimming in honey and upon white bread; he drinks nothing but old muscatel wine."

The King said, "Who has brought these women here, who, all of them, belong to officials of the State?"

She replied, O master of ours, he has in his service an old woman who has had the run of the houses in the town; she chooses and brings to him any woman of superior beauty and perfection; but she serves him only against good consideration in silver, dresses, etc., precious stones, rubies, and other objects of value."

And when does the Negro get that silver?" asked the King. The lady remaining silent, he added "Give me some information, please."

She signified with a sign for the corner of her eye that he had got it all from the wife of the Grand Vizir.

The King understood her, and continued, "O Beder el Bedour! I have faith and confidence in you, and your testimony will have in my eyes the value of that of the two Adels. Speak to me without reserve as to what concerns yourself."

She answered him, "I have not been touched, and however long this might have lasted the Negro would not have had his desire satisfied."

The weird woman

I purchased the Cretan girl, Helena, in a slave-market in Cairo. She was about twenty at the time. Helena (who later converted to Islam, assumed a suitable name, and lived the life of a true believer) was not particularly slim – the opposite in fact – but her skin was smooth and white, her eyes green, and she was not unattractive. I married her when she fell pregnant the first time (altogether she gave me three sons). She clasped me to her during her orgasms, wriggled around under me, rhythmically moving her thighs together and apart, and would mutter things in Greek. When I later desired to know what she had said, she replied that she did not remember any of her words or actions during her moments of bliss.

She was unique in her lovemaking in that her orgasms would cause her vagina to contract tightly and hurt my organ for a moment, until it relaxed again. Her passion was weird and wonderful, and she was lost in her adoration for me.

The Fountains of Pleasure

"Is this so?" asked the King.

She replied, "It is so!" She had understood what the King wanted to say, and the King had seized the meaning of her words.

"Has the negro respected my honor? Inform me about that, said the King.

She answered, "He has respected your honor as far as your wives are concerned. He has not pushed his criminal deeds that far; but if God had spared his days there is no certainty that he would not have tried to soil what he should have respected."

The King having asked her then who those negroes were, she answered, "They are his companions. After he had quite surfeited himself with the women he had caused to be brought to him, he handed them over to them, as you have seen. If it were not for the protection of a woman, where would that man be?"

Then spoke the King, "O Beder el Bedour, why did not your husband ask my help against this oppression? Why did you not complain?"

She replied, "O King of the time, O beloved Sultan, O mater of numerous armies and allies! As regards my husband, I was so far unable to inform him of my lot; as to myself I have nothing to say but what you know by the verses I sang just now. I have given advice to men about women from the first verse to the last."

The King said, "O Beder el Bedour! I like you, I have put the question to you in the name of the chosen Prophet (the benediction and mercy of God be with him!). Inform me of everything; you have nothing to fear; I give you the aman complete. Has this Negro not enjoyed you? For I presume that none of you were out of reach of his attempts and had her honor safe."

She replied, "O King of our time, in the name of your high rank and your power! Look! He, about whom you ask me, O would not have accepted him as a legitimate husband; how could I have consented to grant him the favor of an illicit lover?"

The King said, "You appear to be sincere, but the verses I heard you sing have roused doubts in my soul."

She replied, "I had three motives for employing that language. Firstly, I was at that moment in heat, like a young mare; secondly, Eblis had excited my natural parts; and lastly, I wanted to quiet the Negro and make him have patience, so that he should grant me some delay and leave me in peace until God would deliver me of him."

The King said, "Do you speak seriously?" She was silent. Then the King cried, "O Beder el Bedour, you alone shall be pardoned!" She understood that it was she only that the King would spare from the punishment of death. He then cautioned her that she must keep the secret, and said he wanted to leave now.

Then all the women and virgins approached Beder el Bedour and implored her, saying, "Intercede for us, for you have power over the King;" and they shed tears over her hands, and in despair threw themselves down.

Beder el Bedour then called the King back, as he was going, and said to him, "O our master! You have not granted me any favor yet." "How," said he, "I have sent for a beautiful mule for you; you will mount her and come with us. As for these women, they must all of them die."

She then said, "O our master! I ask you and conjure you to authorize me to make a stipulation which you will accept." The King made oath that he would fulfil it. Then she said, "I ask as a gift the pardon of all these women and of all these maidens. Their deaths would moreover throw the most terrible consternation over the whole town."

The King said, "There is no might nor power but in God, the merciful!" He then ordered the Negroes to be taken out and beheaded. The only exception he made was with the Negro Dorérame, who was enormously stout and had a neck like a bull. They cut off his ears, nose and lips; likewise his virile member, which they put into his mouth, and then hung him on a gallows.

Then the King ordered the seven doors of the house to be closed, and returned to his palace.

The insatiable woman

I met and married the twenty-two-year-old widow, Hafeezah, in her father's house. He was a physician I knew from my days in Samarkand. Hafeezah was still dressed in her widow's garments, since it was only a year since her husband's death. However, her sensual and passionate nature radiated out from those drab garments, and I took a great fancy to her. Within a week, we were married.

I soon discovered that she had a voracious sexual appetite. Far from having to coax her to my bed, she almost knocked me over in her lust.

While her vulva was small, she was blessed with a large clitoris, which quickly – almost upon penetration – led her to extremely intense orgasms, during which she yelped like a dog in pain. She would thrust violently as she approached orgasm, and once it was over, she would slow down, only to resume the wild rhythm and race to the next climax, yelping all the time. This could go on for an hour – with me holding back all the time – and she would climax close to a dozen times. I could not go on for longer than that, and gradually I became tired of her insatiable appetite. She could never get enough, so I divorced her three months later.

The Fountains of Pleasure

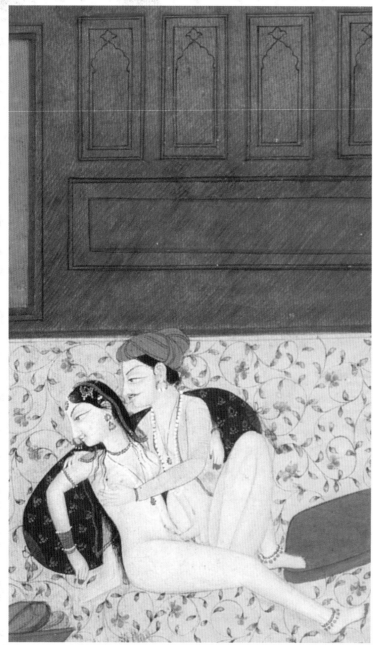

At sunrise he sent a mule to Beder el Bedour, in order to let her be brought to him. He made her dwell with him, and found her to be excelling all those who excel.

Then the King caused the wife of Omar ben Isad to be restored to him, and he made him his private secretary. After which he ordered the Vizir to repudiate his wife. He did not forget the Chaouch and the commander of the Guards, to whom he made large presents, as he had promised, using for that purpose the negro's hoards. He sent the son of his father's Vizir to prison. He also caused the old go-between to be brought before him, and asked her, "Give me all the particulars about the conduct of the Negro, and tell me whether it was well-done to bring in that way women to men." She answered, "This is the trade of nearly all old women." He then had her executed, as well as all old women who followed that trade, and thus cut off in his State the tree of panderism at the root, and burned the trunk.

He besides sent back to their families all the women and girls, and bade them repent in the name of God.

This story presents but a small part of the tricks and stratagems used by women against their husbands.

The moral of the tale is, that a man who falls in love with a woman imperils himself, and exposes himself to the greatest troubles.

The Perfumed Garden of the Sheikh Nefzaoui

About Men Who Are to Be Held in Contempt

Know, O my brother (to whom God be merciful), that a man who is misshapen, of coarse appearance, and whose member is short, thin and flabby, is contemptible in the eyes of women.

When such a man has a bout with a woman, he does not do his business with vigor and in a manner to give her enjoyment. He lays himself down upon her without previous toying, he does not kiss her, nor twine himself around her; he does not bite her, nor such her lips, nor tickle her.

He gets upon her before she has begun to long for pleasure, and then he introduced with infinite trouble a member soft and nerveless. Scarcely has he commenced when he is already done for; he makes one or two movements, and then sinks upon the woman's breast to spend his sperm; and that is the most he can do. This done he withdraws his affair, and makes all haste to get down again from her.

Such a man – as was said by a writer – is quick in ejaculation and slow as to erection; after the trembling, which follows the ejaculation of the seed, his chest is heavy and his sides ache.

Qualities like these are no recommendation with women. Despicable also is the man who is false in his words; who does not fulfill the promise he has made; who never speaks without telling lies, and who conceals from his wife all his doings, expect the adulterous exploits which he commits.

Women cannot esteem such men, as they cannot procure them any enjoyment.

It is said that a man of the mane of Abbes, whose member was extremely small and slight, had a very corpulent wife, whom he could not contrive to satisfy in coition, so that she soon began to complain to her female friends about it.

This woman possessed a considerable fortune, while Abbes was very poor, and when he wanted anything, she was sure not to let him have what he wanted.

One day he went to see a wise man, and submitted his case to him.

The sage told him: "If you had a fine member you might dispose of her fortune. Do you not know that women's religion is in their vulvas? But I will prescribe you a remedy which will do away with your troubles."

Abbes lost no time in making up the remedy according to the recipe of the wise man, and after he had used it his member grew to be long and thick. When his wife saw it in that state she was surprised; but it was still better when he made her feel in the mater of enjoyment quite another thing than she had been accustomed to experience; he began in fact to work her with his tool in quite a remarkable manner, to such a point that she trembled and signed and sobbed and cried out during the operation.

As soon as the wife found in her husband such eminently good qualities she gave him her fortune, and placed her person and all she had at his disposal.

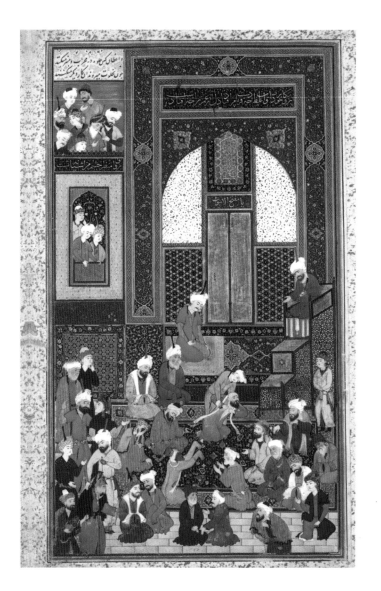

The Perfumed Garden of the Sheikh Nefzaoui

Chapter 4

About Women Who Are to Be Held in Contempt

Know, O Vizir (to whom God be merciful), that women differ in their natural disposition: there are women who are worthy of all praise; and there are, on the other hand, women who only merit contempt.

The woman who merits the contempt of men is ugly and garrulous; her hair is wooly, her forehead projecting, her eyes are small and blear, her nose is enormous, her lips lead-colored, the mouth large, the cheeks wrinkled and she shows gaps in her teeth; her cheekbones shine purple, and she sports bristles on her chin; her head sits on a meager neck, with very much developed tendons; her shoulders are contracted and her chest is narrow, with flabby pendulous breasts, and her belly is like an empty leather-bottle, with the navel standing out like a heap of stones; her flanks are shaped like arcades; the bones of her spinal column may be counted; there is no flesh upon her croup; her vulva is large and cold.

Finally, such a woman has large knees and feet, big hands and emaciated legs.

A woman with such blemishes can give no pleasure to men in general, and least of all to him who is her husband or who enjoys her favors.

The man who approaches a woman like that with his member in erection will find it presently soft and relaxed, as though he was only close to a beast of burden. May God keep us from a woman of that description!

Contemptible likewise is the woman who is constantly laughing out; for, as it was said by an author, "If you see a woman who is always laughing, fond of gaming and jesting, always running to her neighbors, meddling with matters that are no concern of hers, plaguing her husband with constant complaints, leaguing herself with other women against him, playing the grand lady, accepting gifts from everybody, know that that woman is a whore without shame."

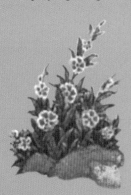

And again to be despised is the woman of a somber, frowning nature, and one who is prolific in talk; the woman who is light-headed in her relations with men, or contentious, or fond of tittle-tattle and unable to keep he husband's secrets, or who is malicious. The woman of a malicious nature talks only to tell lies; if she makes a promise she does so only to break it, and if anybody confides in her, she betrays him; she is debauched, thievish, a scold, course and violent; she cannot give good advice; she is always occupied with the affairs of other people, and with such as to bring harm, and is always on the watch for frivolous news; she is fond of repose, but not of work; she uses unbecoming words

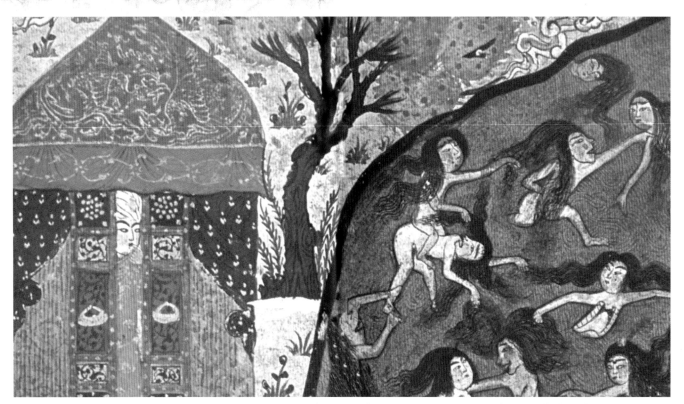

in addressing a Mussulman, even to her husband; invectives are always at her tongue's end; she exhales a bad odor which infects you, and sticks to you even after you have left her.

And not less contemptible is she who talks to no purpose, who is a hypocrite and does no good act; she, who, when her husband asks her to fulfill the conjugal office, refuses to listen to his demand; the woman who does not assist her husband in his affairs; and finally, she who plagues him with unceasing complaints and tears.

A woman of that sort, seeing her husband irritated or in trouble does not share his affliction; on the contrary, she laughs and jests all the more, and does not try to drive away his ill-humor by endearments. She is more prodigal with her person to other men than to her husband; it is not for his sake that she adorns herself, and it is not to please him that she tries to look well. Far from that; with him she is very untidy, and does not mind letting him see things and habits about her person which must be repugnant to him. Lastly, she never uses either atsmed nor souak.

No happiness can be hoped for a man with such a wife. God keep us from such a one!

The Perfumed Garden of the Sheikh Nefzaoui

Chapter 5

Relating to the Act of Generation

Know, O Vizir (and God protect you!), that if you wish for coition, in joining the woman you should not have your stomach loaded with food and drink, only in that condition will your cohabitation be wholesome and good. If you stomach is full, only harm can come of it to both of you will have threatened symptoms of apoplexy and gout, and the least evil that may result from it will be the inability of passing your urine, or weakness of sight.

Let your stomach then be free from excessive food and drink, and you need not apprehend any illness.

Before setting to work with your wife excite her with toying, so that the copulation will finish to your mutual satisfaction.

Thus it will be well to play with her before you introduce your verge and accomplish and cohabitation. You will excite her by kissing her cheeks, sucking her lips and nibbling at her breasts. You will lavish kisses on her navel and thighs, and titillate the lower parts. Bite at her arms, and neglect no part of her body; cling close to her bosom, and show her your love and submission. Interlace your legs with hers, and press her in your arms, for, as the poet has said:

> Under her neck my right hand
> Has served her for a cushion,
> And to draw her to me
> I have sent out my left hand,
> Which bore her up as a bed.

When you are close to a woman, and you see her eyes getting dim, and hear her, yearning for coition, heave deep sighs, then let you're her yearning be joined into one, and let your lubricity rise to the highest point; for this will be the moment most favorable to the game of love. The pleasure which the woman then feels will be extreme; as for yourself, you will cherish her all the more, and she will continue her affection for you, for it has been said:

If you see a woman heaving deep sighs, with her lips getting red and her eyes languishing, when her mouth half opens and her movements grow heedless; when she appears to be disposed to go to sleep, vacillating in her steps and prone to yawn, know that this is the moment for coition; and if you there and then make your way into her you will procure for her an unquestionable treat. You yourself will find the mouth of her womb clasping your article, which is undoubtedly the crowning pleasure for both, for this before everything begets affection and love.

The following precepts, coming from a profound connoisseur in love affairs, are well known:

Woman is like a fruit, which will not yield its sweetness until you rub it between your hands. Look at the basil plant; if you do not rub it warm with your fingers it will not emit any scent. Do you not know that the amber, unless it be handled and warmed, keeps hidden within its pores the aroma contained in it. It is the same with woman. If you do not animate her with your toying, intermixed with kissing, nibbling and touching, you will not obtain from her what you are wishing; you will feel no enjoyment when you share her couch, and you will waken in her heart neither inclination nor affection, nor love for you; all her qualities will remain hidden.

It is reported that a man, having asked a woman what means were the most likely to create affection in the female heart, with respect to the pleasure of coition, received the following answer:

O you who question me, those things which develop the taste for coition are the toyings and touches which precede it, and then the close embrace at the moment of ejaculation!

Believe me, the kisses, nibblings, suction of the lips, the close embrace, the visits of the mouth to the nipples of the bosom, and the sipping of the fresh saliva, these are the things to render affection lasting.

In acting thus, the two orgasms take place simultaneously, and enjoyment comes to the man and woman at the same moment. Then the man feels the womb grasping his member, which gives to each of them the most exquisite pleasure.

This it is which gives birth to love, and if matters have not been managed this way the woman has not had her full share of pleasure, and the delights of the womb are wanting. Know that the woman will not feel her desires satisfied, and will not love her rider unless he is able to act up to her womb; but when the womb is made to enter into action when will feel the most violent love for her cavalier, even if he be unsightly in appearance.

Then do all you can to provoke a simultaneous discharge of the two spermal fluids; herein lies the secret of love.

One of the savants who have occupied themselves with this subject has thus related the confidences which one of them made to him:

O you men, one and all, who are soliciting the love of woman and her affection, and who wish that sentiment in her heart to be of an enduring nature, toy with her previous to coition; prepare her for the enjoyment, and neglect nothing to attain that end. Explore her with the greater assiduity, and, entirely occupied with her, let nothing else engage your thoughts. Do not let the moment propitious for pleasure pass away; that moment will be when you see her eyes humid, half open. Then go to work, but, remember, not till your kisses and toyings have taken effect.

After you have got the woman into a proper state of excitement, O men! Put your member into her, and, if you then observe the proper movements, she will experience a pleasure which will satisfy all her desires.

Lie on her breast, rain kisses on her cheeks, and let not your member quit her vagina. Push for the mouth of her womb. This will crown your labor.

If, by God's favor, you have found this delight, take good care not to withdraw your member, but let it remain there, and imbibe an endless pleasure! Listen to the sighs and heavy breathing of the woman. They witness the violence of the bliss you have given her.

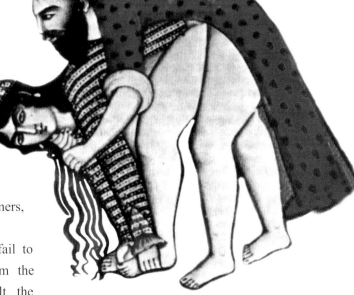

And after the enjoyment is over, and your amorous struggle has come to an end, be careful not to get up at once, but withdraw your member cautiously. Remain close to the woman, and lie down on the right side of the bed that witnessed your enjoyment. You will find this peasant, and you will not be like a fellow who mounts the woman after the fashion of a mule, without any regard to refinement, and who, after the emission, hastens to get his member out and to rise. Avoid such manners, for they rob the woman of all her lasting delight.

In short, the true lover of coition will not fail to observe all that I have recommended; for, from the observance of my recommendations will result the pleasure of the woman, and these rules comprise everything essential in that respect.

God has made everything for the best!

The Perfumed Garden of the Sheikh Nefzaoui

Chapter 6

Concerning Everything that is Favorable to the Act of Coition

Know, O Vizir (God be good to you!) if you would have pleasant coition, which ought to give an equal share of happiness to the two combatants and be satisfactory to both, you must first of all toy with the woman, excite her with kisses, by nibbling and sucking her lips, by caressing her neck and cheeks. Turn her over in the bed, now on her back, now on her stomach, till you see by her eyes that the time for pleasure is near, as I have mentioned in the preceding chapter, and certainly I have not been sparing with my observations thereupon.

Then when you observe the lips of a woman to tremble and get red, and her eyes to become languishing, and her sighs to become quicker, know that she is hot for coition; then get between her thighs, so that your member can enter into her vagina. If you follow my advice, you will enjoy a pleasant embrace, which will give you the greatest satisfaction, and leave with you a delicious remembrance.

Someone has said:

If you desire coition, place the woman on the ground, cling closely to her bosom, with her lips close to yours; then clasp her to you, suck her breath, bite her; kiss her breasts, her stomach, her flanks, press her close in your arms, so as to make her faint with pleasure; when you see her so far gone, then push your member into her. If you have done as I said, the enjoyment will come to both of you simultaneously. That it is which makes the pleasure of the woman so sweet. But if you neglect my advice the woman will not be satisfied and you will not have procured her any pleasure.

The coition being finished, do not get up at once, but come down softly on her right side, and if she has conceived, she will bear a male child, if it pelase God on high!

Sages and Savants (may God grant to all his forgiveness! Have said:

If anyone placing his hand upon the vulva of a woman that is with child pronounces the following words: "In the name of God! May he grant salutation and mercy to his Prophet (salutation and mercy be with him). Oh! My God! I pray to thee in the name of the Prophet to let a boy issue from this conception," it will come to pass by the will of God, and in consideration for our lord Mohammed (the salutation and grace of God be with him), the woman will be delivered of a boy.

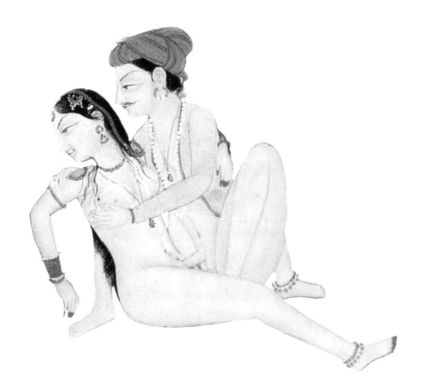

Do not drink rain-water directly after copulation, because this beverage weakens the kidneys.

If you want to repeat the coition, perfume yourself with sweet scents, then close with the woman, and you will arrive at a happy result.

Do not let the woman perform the act of coition mounted upon you, for fear that in that position some drops of her seminal fluid might enter the canal of your verge and cause a sharp urethritis.

Do not work hard directly after coition as this might affect your health adversely, but go to rest for some time.

Do not wash your verge directly after having withdrawn it from the vagina of a woman, until the irritation has gone down somewhat; then wash it and its opening carefully. Otherwise, do not wash your member frequently. Do not leave the vulva directly after the emission, as this may cause canker.

Sundry Positions for the Coitus

The ways of doing it to women are numerous and variable. And now is the time to make known to you the different positions which are usual.

God, the magnificent, has said: "Women are your field. Go upon your field as you like."

According to your wish you can choose the position you like best, provided, of course, that coition takes place in the spot destined for it, that is, in the vulva.

Manner the first – Make the woman lie upon her back, with her thighs raised, then, getting between her legs, introduce your member into her. Pressing your toes to the ground, you can rummage her in a convenient, measured way. This is a good position for a man with a long verge.

Manner the second – If your member is a short one, let the woman lie on he back, lift her legs into the air, so that her right leg be near her right ear, and the left one near her left ear, and in this posture, with her buttocks lifted up, her vulva will project forward. Then put in your member.

Manner the third – Let the woman stretch herself upon the ground, and place yourself between her thighs; then putting one of her legs upon the shoulder, and the other under your arm, near the armpit, get into her.

Manner the fourth – Let her lie down, and put her legs on your shoulders; in this position your member will just face her vulva, which must not touch the ground. And then introduce your member.

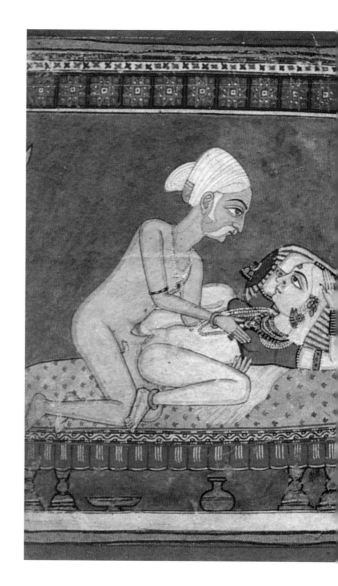

Manner the fifth – Let her lie down on her side, then lie yourself down by her on your side, and getting between her thighs, put your member into her vagina. But sidelong coition predisposes for rheumatic pains and sciatica.

Manner the sixth – Make her get down on her knees and elbows, as if kneeling prayer. In this position the vulva is projected backwards; you then attack her from that side, and put your member into her.

Manner the seventh – Place the woman on her side, and squat between her thighs, with one of her legs on your shoulder and the other between your thighs, while she remains lying on her side. Then you enter her vagina, and make her move by drawing her towards your chest by means of your hands, with which you hold her embraced.

Manner the eighth – Let her stretch herself upon the ground, on her back, with her legs crossed; then mount her like a cavalier on horseback, being on your knees, while her legs are placed under her thighs, and put your member into her vagina.

Manner the ninth – Place the woman so that she leans with her front, or if you prefer it, her back upon a moderate elevation, with her feet set upon the ground. She thus offers her vulva to the introduction of your member.

Manner the tenth – Place the woman near to a low divan, the back of which she can take hold of with her hands; then, getting under her, lift her legs to the height of your navel, and let her clasp you with her legs on each side of your body; in this position plant your verge into her, seizing with your hands the back of the divan. When you begin the action your movements must respond to those of the woman.

Manner the eleventh – Let her lie upon her back on the ground with a cushion under her posterior; then getting between her legs, and letting her place the sole of her right foot against the sole of her left foot, introduce your member.

There are other positions besides the above named in use among the peoples of India. It is well for you to know that the inhabitants of those parts have multiplied the different ways to enjoy women, and they have advanced farther than we in the knowledge and investigation of coitus.

Among those manners are the following, called:

El asemeud, the stopperage
El modefeda, frog fashion
El mokefa, with the toes cramped

El mokeurmeutt, with legs in the air

El setouri, he-goat fashion

El loulabi, the screw of Archimedes

El kelouci, the summersault

Hachou en nekanok, the tail of the ostrich

Lebeuss el djoureb, fitting on the sock

Kechef el astine, reciprocal sight of the posteriors

Neza el kouss, the rainbow arch

Nesedj el Kheuzz, alternative piercing

Dok el arz, pouding on the spot

Nik el kohoul, coition from the back

Et keurchi, belly to belly

Et kebachi, ram-fashion

Dok el outed, driving the peg home

Sebek el heub, love's fusion

Tred ech chate, sheep-fashion

Kalen el miche, interchange in coition

Rekeud el air, the race of the member

El modakheli, the fitter-in

El khouariki, the one who stops in the house

Nik el haddadi, the smith's coition

El moheundi, the seducer

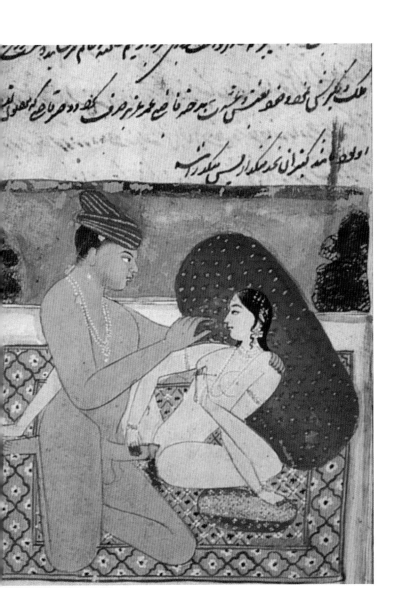

First manner – Et asemeud (the stopperage). Place the woman on her back, with a cushion under her buttocks, then get between her legs, resting the points of your feet against the ground; bend her two thighs against her chest as far as you can; place your hands under her arms so as to enfold her or cramp her shoulders. Then introduce your member, and at the moment of ejaculation draw her towards you. This position is painful for the woman, for her thighs being bent upwards and her buttocks raised by the cushion, the walls of her vagina tighten and the uterus tending forward there is not much room for movement, and scarcely space enough for the intruder; consequently the latter enters with difficulty and strikes against the uterus. This position should therefore not be adopted, unless the man's member is short or soft.

Second manner – Et modefeda (frog fashion). Place the woman on her back, and arrange her thighs so that they touch the heels, which latter are thus coming close to the buttocks; then down you sit in this kind of merry thought, facing the vulva, in which you insert your member; you then place her knees under your armpits; and taking firm hold of the upper part of her arms, you draw her towards you at the crisis.

Third manner – El mokefa (with toes cramped). Place the woman on her back, and squat on your knees as high as your sides, in order that she may cross her legs over your back, and then pass her arms round your neck.

Fourth manner – El mokeurmeutt (with legs in the air). The woman lying on her back, you put her thighs together and raise her legs up until the soles of her feet look at the ceiling; then enfolding her within your thighs you insert your member, holding her legs up with your hands.

Fifth manner – El setouri (he-goat fashion). The woman being crouched on her side, you let her stretch out the leg on which she is resting, and squat down between her thighs with your calves bent under you. Then you lift her uppermost leg so that it rests on your back, and introduce your member. During the action you take hold of her shoulders, or, if you prefer it, her harms.

Sixth manner – El loulabi (the screw of Archimedes). The man being stretched on his back the woman sits on his member, facing him; she then places her hands upon the bed so that she can keep her stomach from touching the man's and moves up and downwards, and if the man is supple he assists her from below. If in this position she wants to kiss him, she need only stretch her arms along the bed.

Seventh manner – El kelouci (the summersault). The woman must wear a pair of pantaloons, which she lets drop upon her heels; then she stoops, placing her head between her feet, so that her neck is in the opening of her pantaloons. At that moment, the man, seizing her legs, turns her upon her back, making her perform a summersault; then with his legs curved under him he brings his member right against her vulva, and, slipping it between her legs, inserts it.

It is alleged that there are women who, while lying on their back, can place their feet behind the head without the help of pantaloons or hands.

Eighth manner – Hachou en nekanok (the tail of the ostrich). The woman lying on her back along the bed, the man kneels in front of her, lifting up her legs until her head and shoulders only are resting on the bed; his member having penetrated into her vagina, he seizes and sets into motion the buttocks of the woman who, on her part, twines her legs around his neck.

Ninth manner – Lebeuss el djoureb (fitting on of the sock). The woman lies on her back. You sit down between her legs and place your member between the lips of her vulva, which you fit over it with your thumb and first finger; then you move so as to procure for your member, as far as it is in contact with the woman, a lively rubbing, which action you continue until her vulva gets moistened with the liquid emitted from your verge. When she is thus amply prepared for enjoyment by the alternative coming and going of your weapon in her scabbard, put it into her in full length.

Tenth manner – Kechef el astine (reciprocal sight of the posteriors). The man lying stretched on his back, the woman sits down upon his member with her back to the man's face, who presses her sides between his thighs and legs, while she places her hands upon the bed as a support for her movements and, lowering her head, her eyes are turned towards the buttocks of the man.

Eleventh manner – Neza el kouss (the rainbow arch). The woman is lying on her side; the man also on his side, with his face towards her back, pushes in between her legs and introduces his member, with his hands lying on the upper part of her back. As to the woman, she then gets hold of the man's feet, which she lifts up as far as she can, drawing him close to her; thus she forms with the body of the man an arch, of which she is the rise.

Twelfth manner – Nesedj el Kheuzz (the alternative movement of piercing). The man in sitting attitude places the soles of his feet together, and lowering his thighs, draws his feet nearer to his member; the woman sits down upon his feet, which he takes care to keep firm together. In this position the two thighs of the woman are pressed against the man's flanks, and she puts her arms round his neck. Then the man clasps the woman's 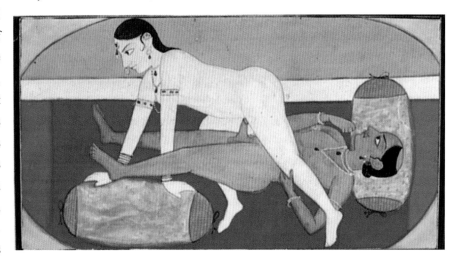 ankles and drawing his feet nearer his body, brings the woman, who is sitting on them, within range of his member, which then enters her vagina. By moving his feet he sends her back and brings her forward again, without ever withdrawing his member entirely.

The woman makes herself as light as possible, and assists as well as she can in this come and go movement; her cooperation is, in fact, indispensable for it. If the man apprehends that his member may come out entirely, he takes her round the waist, and she receives no other impulse than that which is imparted to her by the feet of the man upon which she is sitting.

Thirteenth manner – Dok el arz (pounding on the spot). The man sits down with his legs stretched out; the woman then places herself astride on his thighs, crossing her legs behind the back of the man, and places her vulva opposite his member, which latter she guides into her vagina; she then places her arms round his neck, and he embraces her sides and waist, and helps her to rise and descend upon his verge. She must assist in his work.

Fourteenth manner – Nik el kohoul (coitus from the back). The woman lies down on her stomach and raises her buttocks by help of a cushion; the man approaches from behind, stretches himself on her back and inserts his tool, while the woman twines her arms around the man's elbows. This is the easiest of all methods.

Fifteenth manner – El keurchi (belly to belly). The man and the woman are standing upright, face to face; she opens her thighs; the man then brings his feet forward between those of the woman, who also advances hers a little. In this position the man must have one of his feet somewhat in advance of the other. Each of the two has the arms around the other's hops; the man introduces his verge, and the two move thus intertwined after a manned called Neza el dela, which I shall explain later, if it please God the Almighty (See First movement, page 71)

Sixteenth manner – El kebachi (after the fashion of the ram). The woman is on her knees, with her forearms on the ground; the man approaches from behind, kneels down, and lets his member penetrate into her vagina, which she presses out as much as possible; he will do well in placing his hands on the woman's shoulders.

Seventeenth manner – Dok el outed (driving the peg home). The woman enlaces with her legs the waist of the man, who is standing, with her arms passed around his neck, steadying herself by leaning against the wall. While she is thus suspended the man insinuates his pin into her vulva.

Eighteenth manner – Sebek el heub (love's fusion). While the woman is lying on her right side, extend yourself on your left side; your left leg remains extended, and you raise your right one till it is up to her flank, when you lay her upper leg upon your side thus her uppermost leg serves the woman as a support for her back. After having introduced your member you move as you please, and she responds to your action as she pleases.

Nineteenth manner – Tred ech chate (coitus of the sheep). The woman is on her hands and knees; the man, behind her, lifts her thighs till her vulva is on a level with his member, which he then inserts. In this position she ought to place her head between her arms.

Twentieth manner – Kalen el miche (interchange in coition). The man lies on his back. The woman, gliding in between his legs, places herself upon him with her toenails against the ground; she lifts up the man's thighs, turning them against his own body, so that his virile member faces her vulva, into which she guides it; she then places her hands upon the bed by the sides of the man. It is, however, indispensable that the woman feet rest upon a cushion to enable her to keep her vulva in concordance with his member.

In this position the parts are exchanged, the woman fulfilling that of the man, and vice-versa.

There is a variation to this manner. The man stretches himself out upon his back, while the woman kneels with her legs under her, but between his legs. The remainder conforms exactly to what has been said above.

Twenty-first manner – Bekeud el air (the race of the member). The man, on his back, supports himself with a cushion under his shoulders, but his posterior must retain contact with the bed. Thus placed, he draws up his thighs until his knees are on a level with his face; then the woman sits down, impaling herself on his member; she must not lie down, but keep seated as if on horseback, the saddle being represented by the knees and the stomach of the man. In that position she can, by the play of her knees, work up and down and down and up. She can also pace her knees on the bed, in which case the man accentuates the movement by plying his thighs, while she holds with her left hand on his right shoulder.

Twenty-second manner – El modakheli (the fitter-in). The woman is seated on her coccyx, with only the points of her buttocks touching the ground; the man takes the same position, her vulva facing his member. Then the woman puts her right thigh over the left thigh of the man, while he on his part puts his right thigh over her left one.

The woman, seizing with her hands her partner's arms, gets his member into her vulva; and each of them leaving alternatively a little back, and holding each other by the upper part of the arms, they initiate a swaying movement, moving with little concussions, in keeping their movements in exact rhythm by the assistance of their heels, which are resting on the ground.

Twenty-third manner – El khouriki (the one who stops at home). The woman being couched on her back, the man lies down upon her, with cushions held in his hands.

After his member is in, the woman raises her buttocks as high as she can off the bed, the man following her up with his member well inside, then the woman lowers herself again upon the bed, giving some of the short shocks, and although they do not embrace, the man must stick like glue to her. This movement they continue, but the man must make himself light and must not be ponderous, and the bed must be soft; in default of which the exercise cannot be kept up without break.

Twenty-fourth manner – Nik el haddadi (the coition of the blacksmith). The woman lies on her back with a cushion under her buttocks and her knees raised as far as possible towards her chest, so that her vulva stands out as a target; she then guides her partner's member in.

The man executes for some time the usual action of coition, then draws his tool out of the vulva, and glides it for a moment between the thighs of the woman, as the smith withdraws the glowing iron from the furnace in order to plunge it into cold water. This manner is called sferdgeli, position of quince.

Twenty-fifth manner – El moheundi (the seducer). The woman lying on her back, the man sits between her legs, with his croupe on his feet; then he raises and separates the women's thighs, placing her legs under his arms, or over his shoulders; he then takes her around the waist, or seizes her shoulders.

The preceding descriptions furnish a large number of procedures, that cannot well be all put to the proof; but with such a variety to choose from, the man who finds one of them difficult to practice, can easily find plenty of others more to his convenience.

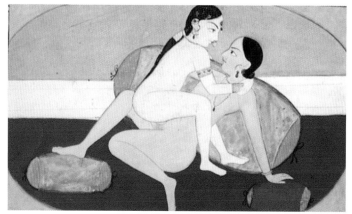

I have not made mention of positions which it appeared to me impossible to realize, and if there be anybody who thinks that those which I have described are not exhaustive, he has only to look for new ones.

It cannot be gainsaid that the Indians have surmounted the greatest difficulties in respect to coition. As a grand exploit, originating with them, the following may be cited:

The woman being stretched out on her back, the man sits down on her chest, with his back turned to her face, his knees turned forward and his nails gripping the ground; he then raises her hips, arching her back until he has brought her vulva face to face with his member, which he then inserts, and thus gains his purpose.

This position, as you perceive, is very fatiguing and very difficult to attain. I even believe that the only realization of it consists in words and designs. With regard to the other methods described above, they can only be practiced if both man and woman are free from physical defects, and of analogous construction; for instance, one or the other of them must not be humpbacked, or very little, or very tall, or too obese. And I repeat, that both must be in perfect health.

I shall now treat of coition between two persons of different conformation. I shall particularize the positions that will suit them in treating each of them severally.

I shall first discourse of the coition of a lean man and a corpulent woman, and the different postures they may assume for the act, assuming the woman to be lying down, and being turned successively over on her four sides.

If the man wants to work her sideways he takes the thigh of the woman which is uppermost, and raises it as high as possible on his flank, so that it rests over his waist; he employs her undermost arm as a pillow for the support of his head, and he takes care to place a stout cushion beneath his undermost hip, so as to elevate his member to the necessary height, which is indispensable on account of the thickness of the woman's thighs.

But if the woman has an enormous abdomen, projecting by reason of its obesity over her thighs and flanks, it will be best to lay her on her back, and to lift up her thighs towards her belly; the man kneels towards him; and if he cannot manage her in consequence of the obesity of her belly and thighs, he must with his two arms encircle her buttocks. But it is thus impossible for him to work her conveniently, owing to the want of mobility of her thighs, which are impeded by her belly. He may, however, support them with his hands, but let him take care not to place them over his own thighs, as, owing to their weight, he would not have the power nor the facility to move. As the poet has said:

If you have to explore her, lift up her buttocks,

In order to work like the rope thrown to a drowning man.

You will then seem between her thighs

Like a rower seated at the end of the boat.

The man can likewise couch the woman on her side, with the undermost leg in front; then he sits down on the thigh of that leg, his member being opposite her vulva, and lets her raise the upper leg, which she must bend at the knee. Then, with his hands seizing her legs and thighs, he introduces his member, with his body lying between her legs, his knees bent, and the points of his feet against the ground, so that he can elevate his posterior, and prevent her thighs from impeding the entrance. In this attitude they can enter into action.

If the woman's belly is enlarged by reason of her being with child, the man lets her lie down on one side; then placing on of her thighs over the other, he raises them both towards the stomach, without their touching the latter; he then lies down behind her on the same side, and can thus fit his member in. In this way he can thrust his took in entirely, particularly by raising his foot, which is under the woman's leg, to the height of her thigh. The same may be done with a barren woman, but it is particularly to be recommended for the woman who is enciente, as the above position offers the advantage of procuring her the pleasure she desires without exposing her to any danger.

In the case of the man being obese, with a very pronounced rotundity of stomach, and the woman being thin, the best course to follow is to let the woman take the active part. To this end, the man lies down on his back with his thighs close together, and the woman lowers herself upon his member, astride of him; she rests her hands upon the bad, and he seizes her arms with his hands. If she knows how to move, she can thus, in turn, rise and sink upon his member; if she is not adroit enough for that movement, the man imparts a movement to her buttocks by the play of one of his thighs behind them. But if the man assumes this position, it may sometimes become prejudicial to him, inasmuch as some of the female sperm may penetrate into his urethra, and grave malady may ensue therefrom. It may also happen – and that is just as bad – that the man's sperm cannot pass out, and returns into the urethra.

If the man prefers that the woman should lie on her back, he places himself, with his legs folded under him, between her legs, which she parts only moderately. Thus, his buttocks are between the woman's legs, with his heels touching them.

In performing this way he will, however, feel fatigue, owing to the position of his stomach resting upon the woman's and the inconvenience resulting therefrom; and, besides, he will not be able to get his whole member in the vulva.

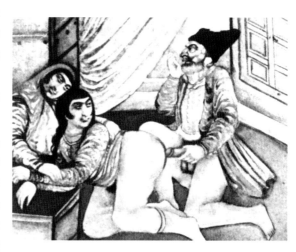

It will be similar when both lie on their sides, as mentioned above in the case of pregnant women.

When both man and woman are fat, and wish to unite in coition, they cannot contrive to do it without trouble, particularly when both have prominent stomachs. In these circumstances the best way to go about it is for the woman to be on her knees with her hands on the ground, so that her posterior is elevated; then the man separates her legs, leaving the points of the feet close together and the heels parted asunder; he then attacks her from behind, kneeling and holding up his stomach with his hand, and so introduces his member. Resting his stomach upon her buttocks during the act he holds the thighs or the waist of the woman with his hands. If her posterior is too low for his stomach to rest upon, he must place a cushion under her knees to remedy this.

I know of no other position so favorable as this for the coition of a fat man with a fat woman.

If, in fact, the man gets between the legs of a woman on her back under the above-named circumstances, his stomach, encountering the woman's thighs, will not allow him to make free use of his tool. He cannot even see her vulva, or only in part; it may be almost said that it will be impossible for him to accomplish the act.

On the other hand, if the man makes the woman lie upon her side, and then places himself, with his legs bent behind her, pressing his stomach upon the upper part of her posterior, she must draw her legs and thighs up to her stomach, in order to lay bare her vagina and allow the introduction of his member; but if she cannot sufficiently bend her knees, the man can either see her vulva, not explore it.

If, however, the stomach of each person is not exaggeratedly large, they can manage very well all positions. Only they must not be too long in coming to the crisis, as they will soon feel fatigued and lose their breath.

In the case of a very big man and a very little woman, the difficulty to be solved is how to contrive that their organs of generation and their mouths can meet at the same time. To gain this end the woman had one of his hands under her neck, and with the other raises her thighs till he can put his member against her vulva from behind, the woman remaining still on her back. In this position he holds her up with his hands by the neck and the thighs. He can then enter her body, while the woman on her part puts her arms around his neck and approaches her lips to his.

If the man wishes the woman to lie on her side, he gets between her legs, and, placing her thighs so that they are in contact with his sides, one above and one under, he glides in between them till his member is facing her vulva from behind; he then presses his thighs against her to them; the other hand he has around her neck. If the man then likes, he can get his thighs over those of the woman, and pres her towards him, this will make it easier for him to move.

As regards the copulation of a very small man and a tall woman, the two actors cannot kiss each other while in action unless they take one of the three following positions, and even then they will become fatigued.

Give back mine eyes their sleep long ravishèd
And say me whither [where] be my reason fled:
I learnt that lending to thy love a place
Sleep to mine eyelids mortal foe was made.
They said, "We held thee righteous, who waylaid
Thy soul?" "Go ask his glorious eyes," I said.
I pardon all my blood he pleased to spill
Owning his troubles drove him blood to shed.
On my mind's mirror sun-like sheen he cast
Whose keen reflection fire in vitals bred
Waters of Life let Allah waste at will
Suffice my wage those lips of dewy red:
An thou address my love thou'lt find a cause
For plant and tears or ruth [sorrow] or lustihed [lustfulness].
In water pure his form shall greet your eyne [eyes]
When fails the bowl nor need ye drink of wine.

The Arabian Nights

First position – The woman lies on her back, with a thick cushion under her buttocks, and a similar one under her head; she then draws up her thighs as far as possible towards her chest. The man lies down upon her, introduces his member, and takes hold of her shoulders, drawing himself up toward them. The woman winds her arms and legs around his back, while he holds on to her shoulders, or if he can, to her neck.

Second position – Man and woman lie both on their side, face to face; the woman slips her undermost thigh under the man's flank, drawing it at the same time higher up; she does the like with her other thigh over his; then she arches her stomach out, while his member is penetrating into her. Both should have hold of the others neck, and the woman, crossing her legs over his back, should draw the man towards her.

Third position – The man lies on his back, with his legs stretched out; the woman sits on his member, and, stretching herself down over him, draws up her knees to the height of her stomach; then, laying her ands over his shoulders, she draws herself up, and presses her lips to his.

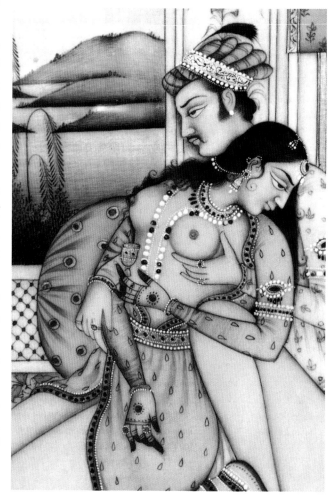

All these postures are more or less fatiguing for both; people can, however, choose any other position they like; but they must be able to kiss each other during the act.

I will now speak to you of those who are little, in consequence of being humpbacked. Of these there are several kinds.

First, there is the man who is crookbacked, but whose spine and neck are straight. For him it is most convenient to unite himself with a little woman, but not otherwise than from behind. Placing himself behind her posterior, he thus introduces his member into her vulva. But if the woman is in as stooping attitude, on her hands and feet, he will do still better. If the woman be afflicted with a hump and the man is straight, the same position is suitable.

If both of them are crookbacked they can take whatever position they like for coition. They cannot, however, embrace; and if they lie on their side, face to face, there will be left an empty space between them. And if one or the other lies down on the back, a cushion must be placed under the head and the shoulder, to hold them up, ad fill the place which is left vacant.

In the case of a man whose malformation affects only his neck, so as to press his chin towards his chest, but who is otherwise straight, he can take any position he likes for ding the business, and give himself up to any embraces and caresses, always excepting kisses on the mouth. If the woman is lying on her back, he will appear in action as if he were butting at her like a ram. If the woman has her neck deformed in similar manner, their coition will resemble the mutual attack of two horned beasts with their heads. The most inconvenient position for them will be that the woman should stoop down, and he attacks her from behind. The man whose hump appears on his back in the shape of only the half of a jar is not so much disfigured as the one of whom the poet has said:

> *Lying on his back he is a dish;*
> *Turn him over, and you have a dish-cover*

In his case coition can take place as with any other man who is small in stature and straight; he cannot, however, easily lie on his back.

If a little woman is lying on her back, with a humpbacked man upon her belly, he will look like the cover over a vase. If, on the contrary, the woman is large-sized, he will have the appearance of a carpenter's plane in action. I have made the following verses on this subject:

> *The humpback is vaulted like an arch*
> *And seeing him you cry, "Glory be to God!"*
> *You ask him how he manages in coitus?*
> *"It is the retribution for my sins," he says.*
> *The woman under him is like a board of deal.*
> *The humpback, who explores her, does the planning.*

I have also said in verse:

> The humpback's dorsal cord is tied in knots,
> The Angels tire with writing all his sins;
> In trying for a wife of proper shape,
> And for her favors, she repulses him,
> And says, "Who bears the wrongs we shall commit?"
> And he, "I bear them well upon my hump!"
> And then she mocks him saying, "Oh, you plane
> Destined for making shavings! Take a deal board!"

If the woman has a hump as well as the man, they may take any of the various positions for coition, always observing that if one of them lies on the back, the hump must be environed with cushion, as with a turban, thus having a nest to lie in, which guards its top, which is very tender. In this way, they can embrace closely.

If the man is humped both on back and chest he must renounce the embrace and the clinging, but can otherwise take any position he lies for coition. Yet generally speaking, the action must always be troublesome for himself and the woman. I have written on this subject:

> The humpback engaged in the act of coition
> Is like a vase provided with two handles.
> If he is burning for a woman, she will tell him,
> "Your hump is in the way; you cannot do it;
> Your verge would find a place to rummage in,
> But on your chest the hump where would it be?"

If both the woman and man have double humps, the best position they can assume for coitus is the following: While the woman is lying on her side, the man introduces his member after the fashion described previously in respect to pregnant women. Thus the two humps do not encounter one another. Both are lying on their sides, and the man attacks from behind. Should the woman be on her back, her hump must be supported by a cushion, while the man kneels between her legs, she loading up her posterior. Thus placed, their two humps are not near each other, and all inconvenience is avoided.

The same is the case if the woman stoops down with her head, with her croup in the air, after the manner of el kouri, which position will suit both of them, if they have the chest malformed, but not the back. One of them then performs the action of come-and-go.

But the most curious and amusing description which I have ever met in this respect, is contained in these verses:

> *Their two extremities are close together,*
> *And nature made a laughing stock of them;*
> *Foreshortened he appears as if cut off;*
> *He looks like someone bending to escape a blow,*
> *Or like a man who has received a blow*
> *And shrivels down so as to miss a second.*

If a man's spine is curved about the hips and his back is straight, so that he looks as though he was in prayer, half prostrated, coition for him is very difficult; owing to the reciprocal positions of his thighs and his stomach, he cannot possibly insert his member entirely, as it lies so far back between his thighs. The best for him to do is to stand up. The woman stoops down before him with her hands to the ground and her posterior in the air; he can thus introduce his member as a pivot for the woman to move upon, for, be it observed, he cannot well move himself. It is the manner el kouri, with the difference, that it is the woman who moves.

A man may be attacked by the illness called ikaad, or zomana (paralysis), which compels him to be constantly seated. If this malady only affects his knees and legs, his thighs and spinal column remaining wound, he can use all the sundry positions for coition, except those where he would have to stand up. In the case of his buttocks being affected, even if he is otherwise perfectly well, it is the woman who will have to make all the movements.

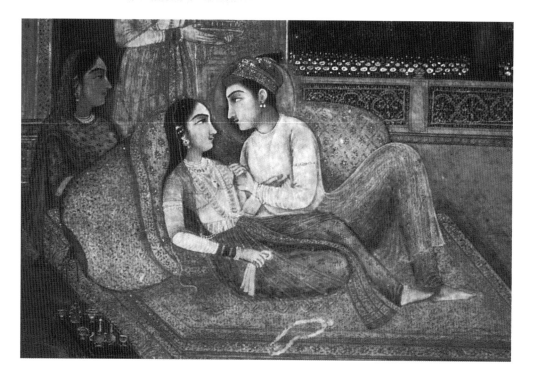

Know that the most enjoyable coitus does not always exist in the manners described here; I only give them, so as to render this work as complete as possible. Sometimes most enjoyable coition takes place between lovers, who, not quite perfect in their proportions, find their own means for their mutual gratification.

It is said that there are women of great experience who, lying with a man, elevate one of their feet vertically in the air, and upon that foot a lamp is set full of oil, and with the wick burning. While the man is ramming them, they keep the lamp steady and burning, and the oil is not spilled. Their coition is in no way impeded by this exhibition, but it must require great previous practice on the part of both.

Assuredly the Indian writers have in their works described a great many ways of making love, but the majority of them do not yield enjoyment, and give more pain than pleasure. That which is to be looked for in coition, the crowning point of it, is the enjoyment, the embrace, the kisses, This is the distinction between the coitus of men and that of animals. No one is indifferent to the enjoyment which proceeds from the difference between the sexes, and the man finds his highest felicity in it.

If the desire of love in man is roused to its highest pitch, all the pleasure of coition becomes easy for him, and he satisfies his yearning in any way.

It is well for the lover of coition to put all these manners to the proof, so as to ascertain which is the position that gives the greatest pleasure to both combatants. Then he will know which to choose for the tryst, and in satisfying his desires retain the woman's affection.

Many people have essayed all the positions I have described, but none has been as much approved of as the dok el arz.

A story is told on this subject of a man who had a wife of incomparable beauty, graceful and accomplished. He used to explore her in the ordinary manner, never having recourse to any other. The woman experienced none of the pleasure which ought to accompany the act, and was consequently generally very moody after the coition was over.

The man complained about this to an old dame, who told him, "Try different ways in united yourself to her, until you find the one which best satisfies her. Then work her in this fashion only, and her affection for you will know no limit."

He then tried upon his wife various manners of coition, and when he came to the one called dok el arz he saw her overcome by violent transports of love, and at the crisis of pleasure he felt her womb grasp his verge energetically; and she said to him, biting his lips, "This is the veritable manner of making love!"

These demonstrations proved to the lover, in fact, that his mistress felt in that position the most lively pleasure, and he always thenceforward worked with her in that way. Thus he attained his end, and caused the woman to love him to folly.

Therefore try different manners; for every woman likes one in preference to all other for her pleasure the majority of them have, however, a predilection for the dok el arz, as, in the application of the same, belly is pressed to belly, mouth glued to mouth, and the action of the womb is rarely absent.

I have now only to mention the various movements practiced during coitus, and shall describe some of them.

First movement – Neza el dela (the bucket in the well). The man and woman join in close embrace after the introduction. Then he gives a push, and withdraws a little; the woman follows him with a push, and also retires. So they continue their alternate movement, keeping proper time. Placing foot against foot, and hand against hand, they keep up the motion of a bucket in a well.

Second movement – El netahi (the mutual shock). After the introduction, they each draw back, but without dislodging the member completely. Then they both push tightly together, and thus go on keeping time.

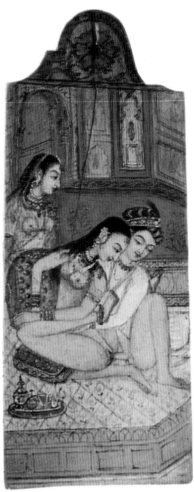

Third movement – El motadani (the approach). The man moves as usual, and then stops. Then the woman, with the member in her receptacle, begins to move like the man, and then stops. And they continue this way until the ejaculation comes.

Fourth Movement – Khiate el heub (love's tailor). The man with his member being only partially inserted in the vulva, keeps up a sort of quick friction with the part that is in, and then suddenly plunges his whole member in up to its root. This is the movement of the needle in the hands of the tailor, of which the man and woman must take cognizance.

Such a movement only suits those men and women who can at will retard the crisis. With those who are otherwise constituted, it would act too quickly.

Fifth movement – Souak el feurdj (the toothpick in the vulva). The man introduces his member between the walls of the vulva, and then drives it up and down, and right and left. Only a man with a very vigorous member can executive this movement.

Sixth movement – Tachik el heub (the boxing up of love). The man introduces his member entirely into the vagina, so closely that his hairs are completely mixed up with the woman's. In that position he must move forcibly, without withdrawing his tool in the least.

This is the best of all the movements, and is particularly well adapted to the positon dok el arz. Women prefer it to any other kind, as it procures them the extreme pleasure of seizing the member with their womb; and appeases their lust most completely.

Those women called tribades always use this movement in their mutual caresses. And it provokes prompt ejaculation both with man and woman.

Without kissing, no kind of position or movement procures the fullest pleasure; and those positions in which the kiss is not practicable are not entirely satisfactory, considering that the kiss is one of the most powerful stimulants to the work of love.

I have said in verse:

> The languishing eye
> Puts in connection soul with soul,
> And the tender kiss
> Takes the message from member to vulva.

The kiss is assumed to be an integral part of coition. The best kiss is the one impressed on humid lips combined with the suction of the lips and tongue, which latter particularly provokes the flow of sweet and fresh saliva. It is for the man to bring this about by slightly and softly nibbling his partner's tongue, when her saliva will flow sweet and exquisite, more pleasant than refined honey, and which will not mix with the saliva of her mouth. This maneuver will give the man a trembling sensation, which will run all through his body, and is more intoxicating than wine drunk to excess.

A poet has said:

> In kissing her, I have drunk from her mouth
> Like a camel that drinks from the redir;
> Her embrace and the freshness of her mouth
> Give me a languor that goes to my marrow.

The kiss should be sonorous; it originates with the tongue touching the palate, lubricated by saliva. It is produced by the movement of the tongue in the mouth and by the displacement of the saliva, provoked by the suction.

The kiss given to the superficial outer part of the lips, and making a noise comparable to the one by which you call your cat, gives no pleasure. It is well enough thus applied to children and hands.

The kiss I have described above is the one for coitus and is full of voluptuousness.

A vulgar proverb says:

> A humid kiss
> Is better than a hurried coitus.

I have composed on this subject the following lines:

You kiss my hand – my mouth should be the place!
O woman, thou who art my idol!
It was a fond kiss you gave me, but it is lost,
The hand cannot appreciate the nature of a kiss.

The three words, kobla, letsem, and bouss are used indifferently to indicate the kiss on the hand or on the mouth. The word ferame means specifically the kiss on the mouth.

An Arab poet has said:

The heart of love can find no remedy
In witching sorcery nor amulets,
Nor in the fond embrace without a kiss,
Nor in a kiss without coitus.

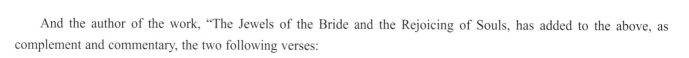

And the author of the work, "The Jewels of the Bride and the Rejoicing of Souls, has added to the above, as complement and commentary, the two following verses:

Nor in converse, however unrestrained,
But in the placing of legs on legs (coition).

Remember that all caresses and all sorts of kisses, as described, are of no account without the introduction of the member. Therefore abstain from the, if you do not want action; they only fan a fire to no purpose. The passion which is excited resembles in fact a fire which is being lighted; and just as water only can extinguish the latter, so only the emission of the sperm can calm the lust and appease the heat.

The woman is not more advantaged than the man by caresses without coition.

It is said that Dahama bent Mesedjel appeared before the Governor of the province of Yamama, with her father and her husband, El Adjadje, alleging that the latter was impotent, and did not cohabit with her nor come near her.

Her father, who assited her in her case, was preproached for mixing himself up with her plaint by the people of Yamama, who said to him, "Are you not ashamed to help your daughter in bringing a claim for coition?"

To which he answered, "It is my wish that she should have children if she loses them it will be by God's will; if she brings them up they will be useful to her."

Dahama formulated her claim thus in coming before the Governor: "There stands my husband, and until now he has never touched me," The Governmore interposed, saying, "No doubt this is because you have been unwilling?" "on the contrary, she replied, "it is for him that I open my thighs and lie down on my back." Then cried the husband, "O Emir, she tells untruth, in order to possess her I have to fight with her." The time to prove her allegaton to be false." He decided thus out of regard for the man. El Adjadje then went away reciting those verses:

> *Dahama and her father Mesedjel thought*
> *The Emir would decide upon my impotence.*
> *Is not the stallion sometimes lazyominded?*
> *And yet his is so large and vigorous.*

Returned to his house he began to kiss and caress his wife; but his efforts went no father, he remained incapable of giving proof of his virility. Dahama said to him, "Keep your caresses and embraces; they do not satisfy love. What I desire is a solid and stiff member, the sperm of which will flow into my matrix." And she recited to him the following verses:

> *Before God! It is in vain to try with kisses*
> *To entertain me, and with your embracings!*
> *To still my torments I must feel a member,*
> *Ejaculating sperm into my uterus.*

El adjadje, in despair, conducted her forthwith back to her family, and, to hid his shame, repudiated her that very night.

A poet said on that occasion:

What are caresses to an ardent woman,
Or costly refreshments and fine jewelry,
If the man's organs do not meet her own,
And she is yearning for the virile verge?

Know then that the majority of women do not find full satisfaction in kisses and embraces without coition. For them satisfaction resides only in the member, and they like the man who rummages them, even if he is ugly and misshapen.

A story also goes on this subject that Moussa ben Mesab betook himself one day to a woman in the town who had a female slave, an excellent singer, whom he wanted to buy from her. This woman was resplendently beautiful, and independent of her charming appearance, she had a large fortune. He saw at the same time in the house a young man of bad shape and ungainly appearance, who went to and fro giving orders.

Moussa asked who the man was, she told him, "This is my husband, and for him I would give my life!" "This is a hard slavery," he said, to which you are reduced, and I am sorry for you. We belong to God, and shall return to him but what a misfortune it is that such incomparable beauty and such delightful forms as I see in you should be for such a man!"

She made answer, "O son of my mother, if he could do to you from behind what he does for me in front, you would sell your lately acquired fortune as well as your patrimony. He would appear to you beautiful, and his plain looks would be changed into beauty."

"May God preserve him to you!" said Moussa.

It is also said that the poet Farazdak met one day a woman on whom he cast a glance burning with love, and who for that reason thus addressed him: "What makes you look at me in this fashion? Had I a thousand vulvas, there would be nothing to hope for for you!" And why?" said the poet. "Because your appearance is not prepossessing," she said, "and what you keep hidden will be no better." He replied, "If you would put me to the proof, you would find that my interior qualities are of a nature to make you forget my outer appearance." He then uncovered himself, and let her see a member

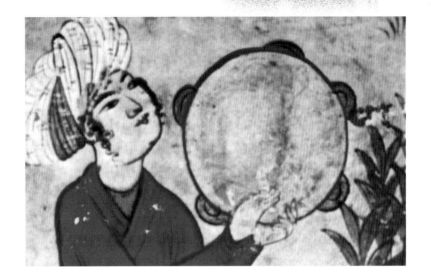

the size of the arm of a young girl. At that sight she felt herself burning hot with amorous desire. He saw this, and asked her to let him caress her. Then she uncovered herself and showed him her mount of Venus, vaulted like a cupola. He then did the business for her, and recited these verses:

I have plied in her my member, big as a virgin's arm;
A member with a round head, and prompt to attack;
Measuring in length a span and a half,
And, oh! I felt as though I had put it in a brazier.

He who seeks the pleasure a woman can give must satisfy her amorous desire for hot caresses, as described. He will see her swooning with lust, her vulva will get moist, her womb will stretch forward, and the two sperms will come together.

The Perfumed Garden of the Sheikh Nefzaoui

The crying woman

Dhabya was the Arabic name I gave to a Frankish captive I purchased in Damascus. She was about twenty, and had been there for a year. She was a tall, shapely woman with long blonde hair and blue eyes, plump red lips and straight white teeth. She barely spoke Arabic, but she was certainly a sight for sore eyes.

While she did not resist when I mounted her, she showed no eagerness either, despite my excitement. On the contrary, she was frigid, and would not allow herself to savor the pleasures of sex. What she could not control, however, was the wetness of her vagina during foreplay. She refused to open her mouth when I kissed her, and any kissing of her lower lips was strictly out of bounds as far as she was concerned.

Some time later, in a state of feverish desire, I decided that I would get her to respond, even if I died while doing so. To this end, I licked and sucked one of her magnificent breast and, keeping it in my mouth, elevated her bottom so that my organ was in constant contact with her clitoris. My thrusts came fast and furious. All of a sudden, I heard a sharp intake of breath. Alarmed, I thought I had inadvertently bitten her nipple. When I looked at her face, I saw that her eyes were wide open, and huge tears were flowing out of them. Then she squeezed them shut, clasped me tightly, and began to respond to my thrusts until she reached orgasm, sobbing and crying all the while. Her orgasm, which lasted well over thirty seconds – I have never seen a woman have such a long orgasm – subsided very slowly. Afterwards, when I wanted to kiss her, she permitted me to place my tongue in it, but soon turned over and fell asleep.

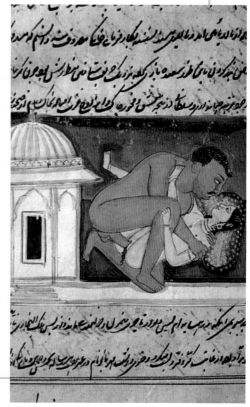

After that, she always reached orgasm when we had intercourse, but it was never as long and as intense as the first time. Her habit of crying and sobbing endured, however, but I never knew the reason for it – whether it reminded her of someone she had loved and lost, or whether the sheer depth of her pleasure caused her to weep. She did not last long, unfortunately – she fell ill and died a year later.

The Fountains of Pleasure

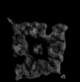
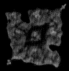

Chapter 7

Of Matter Which are Injurious in the Act of Generation

Know, O

(to whom God be good!) that the ills caused by coition are numerous. I will mention to you some of them, which to know is essential in order to be able to avoid them.

Let me tell you in the first place that coition if performed standing affects the knee-joints and brings about nervous shiverings; and if performed sideways will predispose your system for gout and sciatica, which resides chiefly in the hip joint.

Do not mount upon a woman fasting or immediately before making a meal, or else you will have pains in your back, you will lose your vigor, and your eyesight will get weaker.

If you do it with the woman bestriding you, your dorsal cord will suffer and your heart will be affected; and if in that position the smallest drop of the usual secretions of the vagina enters your urethral canal, a painful stricture may supervene.

Do not leave your member in the vulva after ejaculation, as this might cause gravel, or softening of the vertebral column, or the rupture of blood vessels or, lastly, inflammation of the lungs.

Too much exercise after coition is also detrimental.

Avoid washing your member after the copulation, as this may cause canker.

As to coition with old women, it acts like a fatal poison, and it has been said, "Do not rummage old women, were they as rich as Karoun." And it has further been said, "Beware of mounting old women; even if they cover you with favors." And again, "The coitus of old women is a venomous meal."

Know that the man who works a woman younger than he is himself acquires new vigor; if she is of the same age as he is he will derive no advantage from it; and, finally, if it is a woman older than himself she will take all his strength out of him for herself. The following verses treat on this subject:

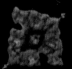

Be on your guard and shun coition with old women;

In her bosom she bears the poison of the arakime.

A proverb says also,

"Do not serve an old woman, even if she offered to feed you with semolina and almond bread."

The excessive practice of coition injures the health on account of the expenditure of too much sperm. For as butter made of cream represents the quintessence of the milk, and if you take the cream off, the milk loses its qualities, even so does the sperm form the quintessence of nutrition, and its loss is debilitating. On the other hand, the condition of the body, and consequently the quality of the sperm depends directly upon the food you take. If, therefore, a man will passionately give himself up to the enjoyment of coition, without undergoing too great fatigue, he must live upon strengthening food, exciting comfits, aromatic plants, meat, honey, eggs, and other similar viands. He who follows such a regime is protected against the following accidents, to which excessive coition may lead.

Firstly, the loss of generative power.

Secondly, the deterioration of his sight; for although he may not become blind, he will at least have to suffer from eye diseases if he does not follow my advice.

Thirdly, the loss of his physical strength; he may become like the man who wants to fly but cannot, who pursuing somebody cannot catch him, or who carrying a burden, or working, soon gets tired and prostrated.

He who does not want to feel the necessity for coition uses camphor. Half of a mitskal of this substance, macerated in water, makes the man who drinks of it insensible to the pleasures of copulation. Many women use this remedy when in fits of jealousy against rivals, or when they need repose after great excesses. Then they try to procure camphor that has been left after a burial, and shrink from no expense of money to get such from the old women who have the charge of the corpses. They also make use of the flower of henna, which is called faria, they macerate the same in water, until it turns yellow, and thus supply themselves with a beverage which has almost the same effect as camphor.

I have treated of these remedies in the present chapter, although this is not their proper place; but I thought that this information, as here given, may be of use to many persons.

There are certain things which will become injurious if constantly indulged in and which in the end affect the health. Such are: too much sleep, long voyages in unfavorable season, which latter, particularly in cold countries, may weaken the body and cause disease of the spine. The same effects may arise from the habitual handling of those bodies which engender cold and humidity, like plaster, etc.

For people who have difficulty in passing water, coitus is hurtful. The habit of consuming acid food is debilitating.

To keep one's member in the vulva of a woman after ejaculation has taken place, be it for a long or a short time, enfeebles that organ and makes it less fit for coition.

If you are lying with a woman, do her business several times if you feel inclined, but take care not to overdo it, for it is a true work that, "He who plays the game of love for his own sake, and to satisfy his desires, feels the most intense and durable pleasure; but he who does it to satisfy the lust of another person will languish, lose all his desire, and finish by becoming impotent for coition."

The sense of these words is, that a man when he feels disposed for it can give himself up to the exercise of coitus with more or less ardor according to his desires, and at the time which best suits him, without any fear of future impotence, if his enjoyment is provoked and regulated only by his feeling with want of lying with a woman.

But he who makes love for the sake of somebody else, that is to say only to satisfy the passion of his mistress, and tries all he can to attain that impossibility, that man will act against his own interest and imperil his health to please another person.

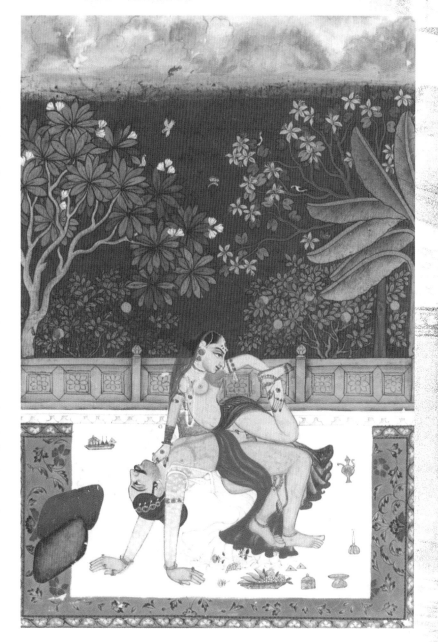

As injurious may be considered coition in the bath or immediately after leaving the bath; after having been bled or purged or suchlike. Coitus after a heavy bout of drinking is likewise to be avoided. To indulge in coitus with a woman during her courses is as detrimental to the man as to the woman herself, as at that time her blood is vitiated and her womb cold, and if the least drop of blood should get in the man's urinary canal numerous maladies may supervene. As to the woman, she feels no pleasure during her courses, and at such time holds coitus in aversion.

As regards copulation in the bath, some say that there is no pleasure to be derived from it, if as it is believed, the degree of enjoyment is dependent upon the warmth of the vulva; for in the bath the vulva cannot be otherwise than cold, and consequently unfit for giving pleasure. And it is besides not to be forgotten that the water penetrating into the sexual parts of man or woman may lead to grave consequences.

Coitus after a full mean may occasionally rupture the intestines. It is also bee be avoided after undergoing much fatigue, or at a time of very hot or very cold weather.

Among the accidents which may attend the act of coition in the countries may be mentioned sudden blindness without any previous symptoms.

The repetition of the coitus without washing the parts ought to be shunned, as it may enfeeble the virile power.

The man must also abstain from copulation with his wife if he is in a state of legal impurity, for if she should become pregnant by such coition, the child could not be sound.

After ejaculation do not remain close to the woman, as the disposition for recommencing will suffer by doing so.

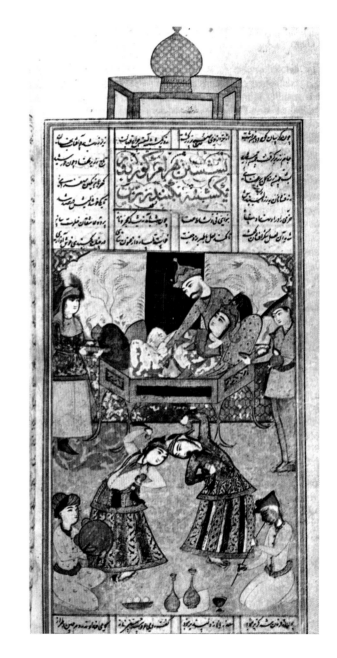

Care is to be taken not to carry heavy loads on one's back or to over-exert the mind, if one does not want the coitus to be impeded. It is also not good constantly to wear vestments made of silk, as they impair all the energy for copulation.

Silken cloths worn by women also affect injuriously the capacity for erection of the virile member.

Fasting, if prolonged, calms sexual desire; but in the beginning it excites the same.

Abstain from greasy liquids, as in the course of time they diminish the strength necessary for coition.

The effect of snuff, whether plain or scented, is similar.

It is bad to wash the sexual parts with cold water directly after copulation; in general, washing with cold water calms down the desire, while warm water strengthens it.

Conversation with a young woman excites in a man the erection and passion commensurate with the youthfulness of the woman.

An Arab addressed the following recommendation to his daughter at the time when he conducted her to her husband: "Perfume yourself with water!" meaning that she should frequently wash her body with water in preference to perfumes; the latter, moreover, not being suitable for everyone.

It is also reported a woman having said to her husband, "You are then a nobody, as you never perfume yourself!" he made answer, "Oh, you sloven! It is for the woman to emit a sweet odor."

The abuse of coition is followed by loss of the taste for its pleasures; and to remedy this loss the sufferer must anoint his member with a mixture of the blood of a he-goat with honey. This will procure for him a marvelous effect in making love.

It is said that reading the Koran also predisposes for copulation.

Remember that a prudent man will beware of abusing the enjoyment of coition. The sperm is the water of life; if you use it economically you will always be ready for love's pleasure; it is the light of your eye; do not be lavish with it at all times and whenever you have a fancy for enjoyment, for if you are not sparing with it you will expose yourself to many ills. Wise medical men say, "A robust constitution is indispensable for copulation, and he who is endowed with it may give himself up to the pleasure without danger; but it is otherwise with the weakly man; he runs into danger by indulging feely with women."

The sage, Es Sakli, has thus determined the limits to be observed by man as to the indulgence of the pleasure of coition: Man, be he phlegmatic or sanguine, should not make love more than twice of thrice a month; bilious or hypochondriac men only once or twice a month. It is nevertheless a well-established fact that nowadays men of any of these four temperaments are insatiable as to coition, and give themselves up to it day and night, taking no heed how they expose themselves to numerous ills, both internal and external.

Women are more favored than men in indulging their passion for coition. It is in fact their specialty; and for them it is all pleasure; while men run many risks in abandoning themselves without reserve to the pleasures of love.

Having thus been treated of the dangers which may occur from the coitus, I have considered it useful to bring to your knowledge the following verses, which contain hygienic advice in their respect. These verses were composed by the order of Haroun er Rachid by the most celebrated physicians of his time, whom he had asked to inform him of the remedies for successfully combating the ills caused by coition.

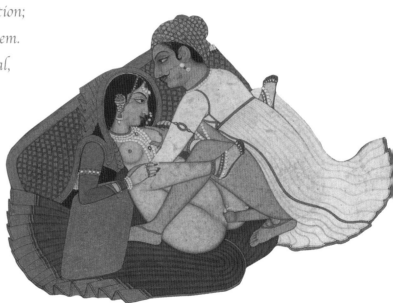

Eat slowly, if your food shall do you good,
And take good care, that it be well-digested.
Beware of things which want hard mastication;
They are bad nourishment, so keep from them.
Drink not directly after finishing your meal,
Or else you go half way to meet an illness.
Keep not within you what is of excess.
And if you were in most susceptible circles,
Attend to this well before seeking your bed,
For rest this is the first necessity.
From medicines and drugs keep well away,
And do not use them unless very ill.
Use all precautions proper, for they keep
Your body sound, and are the best support.
Don't be too eager for round-breasted women;
Excess of pleasure soon will make you feeble,
And in coition you may find a sickness;
And then you find too late that in coition

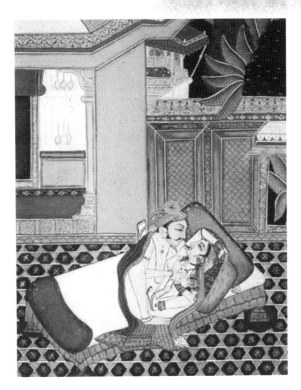

Our spring of life runs into woman's vulva.
And before all beware of aged women,
For their embraces will to you be poison.
Each second day a bath should wash you clean;
Remember these precepts and follow them.

Those were the rules given by the sages to the master of benevolence and goodness, to the generous of the generous.

All sages and physicians agree in saying that the ills which afflict man originate with the abuse of coition. The man therefore who wishes to preserve his health, and particularly his sight, and who wants to lead a pleasant life, will indulge with moderation in love's pleasure, aware that the greatest evils may spring therefrom.

The Perfumed Garden of the Sheikh Nefzaoui

Chapter 8

The Sundry Names Given to the Sexual Parts of Man

Know, O Vizir (to whom God be good!), that man's member bears different names, as:

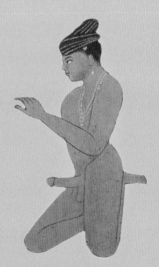

El dekeur, the virile member

El kamera, the penis

El air, the member for generation

El hamama, the pigeon

El teunnana, the tinkler

El heurmak, the indomitable

El ahlil, the liberator

El zeub, the verge

El hammache, the exciter

El naasse, the sleeper

El zodamme, the crowbar

El khiade, the tailor

Mochefi el relil, the extinguisher of passion

El khorate, the turnabout

El deukkak, the striker

El aouame, the swimmer

El dekhal, the housebreaker

El aouar, the one-eyed

El fortass, the bald one

Abou ame, he with one eye

El atsar, the pusher

El dommar, the odd-headed

Abou rokba, the one with a neck

Abou quetaia, the hairy one

El besiss, the impudent one

El mostahi, the shame-faced one

El bekkai, the weeping one

El hezzas, the rummager

El lezzas, the unionist

Abou laaba, the expectorant

El fattache, the searcher

El hakkak, the rubber

El mourekhi, the blabby one

El motela, the ransacker

El moksheuf, the discoverer

As regards the names of kamera and dekeur, their meaning is plain. Dekeur is a word which signifies the male of all creatures, and is also used in the sense of mention and memory. When a man has met with an accident to his member, when it has been amputated, or has become weak, and he can, in consequence, no longer fulfill his conjugal duties, they say of him: "the member of such a one is dead;"which means: the remembrance of him will be lost, and his generation is cut off by the root. When he dies they will say, "His member has been cut of," meaning, "His memory is departed from the world."

The dekeur plays also an important part in dreams. The man who dreams that his member has been cut off is certain not to live long after that dream, for as said above, it presages the loss of his memory and the extinction of his race.

I shall treat this subject more particularly in the explication of dreams.

The teeth (senane) represent years (senine); if therefore a man sees in a dream a fine set of teeth, this is for him the sign of a long life.

If he sees his nail (defeur) reversed or upside down, this is an indication that the victory (defeur) which he has gained over this enemies will change sides; and from a victor, he will become the vanquished; inversely, if he sees the nail of his enemy turned the wrong way, he can conclude that the victory which has been with his enemy will soon return to him.

> *On her fair bosom caskets twain [two] I scanned [noticed],*
> *Scaled fast with musk-seals lovers to withstand;*
> *With arrowy glances stand on guard her eyes,*
> *Whose shafts would shoot who dares put forth a hand.*
>
> *The Arabian Nights*

The sight of a lily (sonsana) is the prognostication of a misfortune which will last a year (son, misfortune; sena, year).

The appearance of ostriches (namate) in dreams is of bad augury, because their name being formed of naa and mate, signifies "news of death," namely, peril.

To dream of a shield (henafa) means the coming on of all sorts of misfortune, for this word, by a change of letters, gives koul afa, "all bad luck."

The sight of a fresh rose (ouarde) announces the arrival (ouraud) of a pleasure to make the heart tremble with joy; while a faded rose indicated deceitful news. It is the same with baldness of the temples, and similar things

The jessamine (yasmine) is formed of yas, signifying deception, or the happening of a thing contrary to your wish, and mine, which means untruth. The man, then, who sees a jessamine in his dream is to conclude that the deception, yas, in the name yasmine, is an untruth, and will thus be assured of the success of his enterprise. However, the prognostications furnished by the jessamine have not the same character of certainty as those given by the rose. It differs, in fact, greatly from this latter flower, inasmuch as the slightest breath of wind will upset it.

The sight of a saucepan (beurma) announces the conclusion (anuberame) or affairs in which one is engaged. Abou Djahel (God's curse be upon him!) has added that such conclusion would take place during the night.

A jab (khabia) is the sign of turpitude (khebets) in every kind of affair, unless it is one that has fallen into a pit or a river and got broken, so as to let escape all the calamities contained in it.

The swing of wood (nechara) means good news (bechara).

The inkstand (douaia) indicates the remedy (doua), namely, the cure of a malady, unless it be burnts, broken or lost, when it means the contrary.

The turban (amama) if seen to fall over the face and cover the eyes is a presage of blindness (aina), from which God preserve us!

The finding again in good condition a gem that has been lost of forgotten is a sign of success.

If one dreams that he gets out of a window (taga) he may know that he will come with advantage out of all transactions he may have, whether important or not. But if the window seen in the dream is narrow so that he had some trouble to get out of it, this will be to him a sign that in order to be successful he will have to make efforts in proportion to the difficulty experienced by him in getting out.

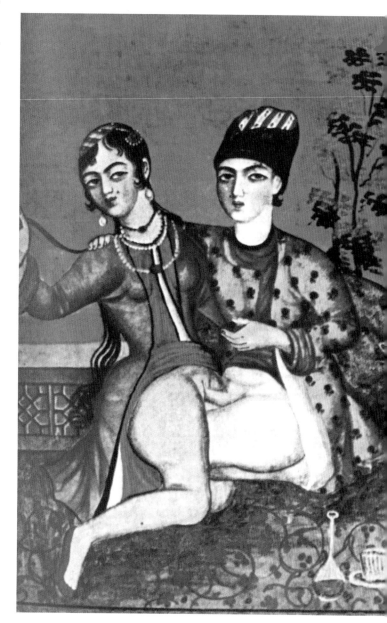

The bitter orange signifies that from the place where it was seen calumnies will be issuing.

Trees (achedjar) means discussions (mechadjera).

The carrot (asafnaria) prognosticates misfortune (asef) and sorrow.

The turnip (cufte) means for the man that has seen it a matter that is past and gone (ameur fate), so that there is no going back to it. The matter is weighty if it appeared large, of no importance if seen small; in short, important in proportion to the size of the turnip that has been seen.

A musket seen without its being fired means a complot contrived in secret, and of no importance. But if it is seen going off it is a sign that the moment has arrived for the realization of the complot.

The sight of fire is of bad augury.

If the pitcher (brik) of a man who has turned to God breaks, this is a sign that his repentance is in vain, but if the glass out of which drinks wine breaks, this means that he returns to God.

If you have dreamed of feasts and sumptuous banquets, be sure that quite contrary things will come to pass.

If you have seen somebody bidding adieu to people on their going away you may be certain that it will be the latter who will shortly wish him a good journey; for the poet says:

If you have seen your friend saying goodbye, rejoice;
Let your soul be content as to him who is far away,
For you may look forward to his speedy return,
And the heart of him who said adieu will come back to you.

The coriander (keusbeur) signifies that the vulva (keuss) is in proper condition.

On this subject there is a story that the Sultan Haroun er Rachid, having with him several persons of mark with whom he was familiar, rose and left them to go to one of his wives, whom he wanted to enjoy. He found her suffering from her courses, and returned to his companions to sit down with them, resigned to his disappointment.

Now it so happened that a moment afterwards the woman found herself free from her discharge. When she had assured herself of this she made forthwith her ablutions, and sent to the Sultan, by one of her negresses, a plate of coriander.

Haround er Rachid was seated among his friends when the negress brought the plate to him. He took it and examined it, but did not understand the meaning of its being sent to him by his wife. At last he handed it to one of his poets, who, having looked at it attentively, recited to him the following verses:

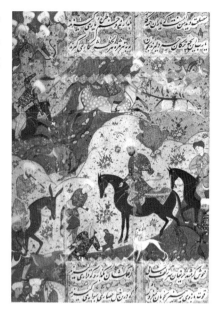

> *"She has sent you coriander*
> *White as sugar;*
> *I have placed it in my palm,*
> *And concentrated all my thoughts upon it,*
> *In order to find out its meaning;*
> *And I have seized it. O my master, what she wants to say,*
> *Is, 'My vuva is restored to health.'"*

Er Rachid was surprised at the wit shown by the woman, and at the poet's penetration. Thus that which was to remain a mystery remained hidden, and that which was to be known was divulged.

A drawn sword is a sign of war, and the victory will remain with his who holds its hilt.

A bridle means servitude and oppression.

A long beard points to good fortune and prosperity; but it is said that it is a sign of death if it reaches down to the ground.

Others pretend that the intelligence of each man is in an inverse proportion to the length of his beard; that is to say, a big beard denotes a small mind. A story goes in this respect, that a man who had a long beard saw one day a book with the following sentence inscribed on its back: "He whose chin is garnished with a large beard is as foolish as his beard is long." Afraid of being taken for a fool by his acquaintances, he thought of getting rid of what there was too much of, and to this end, it being a night-time, he grasped a handful of his beard close to the chin, and set the remainder on fire by the light of the lamp. The flame ran rapidly up the beard and reached his hand, which he had to withdraw precipitately on account of the heat. Thus his beard was burnt off entirely. Then he wrote on the back of the book, under the above-mentioned sentence, "These words are entirely true. I, who am now writing this, have proved their truth." Being himself convinced that the weakness of the intellect is proportioned to the length of the beard.

On the same subject it is related that Haroun er Rachid, being in a kiosk, saw a man with a long beard. He ordered a man to be brought before him, and when he was there he asked him, "What is your name?"

"Abou Arouba," replied the man.

What is your profession?"

"I am a master in controversy."

Haroun then gave him the following case to solve. A man buys a he-goat, who, in voiding his excrements, hits the buyer's eye with part of it and injures the same. "Who has to pay for damages?" "The seller," promptly says Abou Arouba. "And why?" asked the Caliph. "Because he has sold the animal without warning the buyer that it has a catapult in its anus," answered the man. At these words the Caliph began to laugh immoderately, and recited the following verses:

> When the beard of the young man
> Has grown down to his navel,
> The shortness of his intellect is, in my eyes,
> Proportioned to the length his beard has grown.

It is averred by many authors that among proper names there are such as bring luck, and others that bring ill luck, according to the meaning they bear.

The names Ahmed, Mohammed, Hamdonna and Hamdoun indicate in encounters and in dreams the lucky issue arrived at in a transaction. Ali and Alia, indicate the height and elevation of rank. Naserouna, Naseur, Mansour and Naseur Allah signify triumph over enemies. Salem, Salema, Selim and Selimane indicate success in all affairs; also security for him who is in danger. Fetah Allah and Fetah indicate victory, like all the other names which in their meaning speak of lucky things. The names Rad And Rada signify thunder, tumult, and comprise everything in connection with this meaning. Abou el Feurdj and Ferendj indicate job; Ranem and Renime success, Khalf Allah and Khaleuf compensation for a loss, and benediction. The sense of Abder Rassi, Hafid and Mahfond is favorable. The names in which are the word latif (benevolent) mourits (helpful), hanine (compassionate) and aziz (beloved), carry with them, in conformity with the sense of these words, the ideas of benevolence, lateuf (charity) iratsa (compassion), hanana, and aiz (favor). As an example of words of an unfavorable omen I will cite el ouar and el auara, which imply the idea of difficulties.

As supporting the truth of the preceding observations I will refer to this saying of the prophet (the salutation and benevolence of God to him!), "Compare the names appearing in your dreams with their signification, so that you may draw therefrom your conclusions."

I must confess that this was not the place for treating of this subject, but one work leads on to more. I now return to the object of this chapter, viz: the different names of the sexual parts of man.

The name of el air is derived from el kir (the smith's bellows). In fact, if you turn in the latter work the k, kef, so that it faces the opposite way, you will find the word to read el air. The member is so called on account of its alternate swelling and subsiding again. If swollen up it stands erect, and if not it sinks down flaccid.

"If Time unite us after absent-while,
The world harsh frowning on our lot shall smile;
And if thy semblance deign adorn mine eyes,
I'll pardon Time past wrongs and by-gone guile."
The Arabian Nights

It is called *el hamama* (the pigeon), because after having been swelled out it resembles at the moment when it returns to repose a pigeon sitting on her eggs.

El teunnana (the tinkler) – So called because every time it enters or comes out of the vulva in coition it makes a noise.

El heurmak (the indomitable) – It has received this name because when in a state of erection it begins to move its head, searching for the entrance to the vulva till it has found it, and it then walks in quite insolently, without asking leave.

El ahlil (the liberator) – Thus called because in penetrating into the vulva of a woman thrice repudiated it gives her the liberty to return to her first husband.

El zeub (the verge) – From the word deub, which means creeping. This name was given to the member because when it gets between a woman's thighs and feels a plump vulva it begins to creep upon the thighs and the Mount of Venus, then approaches the entrance of the vulva, and keeps creeping in until it is in possession and is comfortably lodged, and having it all its own way penetrates into the middle of the vulva, there to ejaculate.

El hammache (the exciter) – It has received this name because it irritates the vulva by its frequent entries and exits.

El naasse (the sleeper) – From its deceitful appearance. When it gets into erection, it lengthens out and stiffens itself to such an extent that one might think it would never get soft again. But when it has left the vulva, after having satisfied its passion, it goes to sleep.

There are members that fall asleep while inside the vulva, but the majority of them come out still firm; but at that moment they get drowsy, and little by little they go to sleep.

El zoddame (the crowbar) – It is called so because when it meets the vulva and the same will not let it pass in directly, it forces the entrance with its head, breaking and tearing everything, like a wild beast in the rutting season.

El Khiade (the tailor) – It takes this name from the circumstance that it does not enter the vulva until it has maneuvered about the entrance, like a needle in the hand of a tailor, creeping and rubbing against it until it is sufficiently roused, after which it enters.

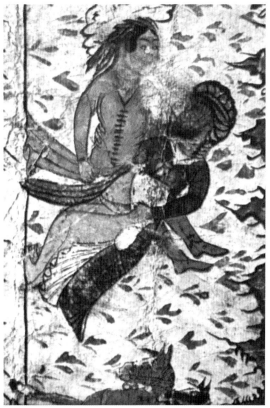

Mochefi el relil (the extinguisher of passion) – This name is given to a member which is large, strong, and slow to ejaculate; such a member satisfies most completely the amorous wishes of a woman; for, after having wrought her up to the highest pitch, it allays her excitement better than any other. And, in the same way, it calms the ardor of the man. When it wants to get into the vulva, and arriving at the portal finds it closed, it laments, begs and promises: "Oh! My love! Let me come in, I will not stay long." And when it has been admitted, it breaks its word and makes a long stay, and does not take its leave till it has satisfied its ardor by the ejaculation of the sperm, coming and going, tilting high and low, and rummaging right and left. The vulva protests, "How about your word, you deceiver?" she says; "you said you would only stop in for a moment." And the member answers, "Oh, certainly! I shall not retire till have encountered your womb; but after having found it, I will engage to withdraw at once." At these words, the vulva takes pity on him, and advances her matrix, which clasps and kisses its head, as if saluting it. The member then retires with its passion cooled down.

El khorrate (the turnabout) – This name was given to it because on arriving at the vulva it pretends to come on important business, knocks at the door, turns about everywhere, without shame or bashfulness, investigating every corner to the right and left, forward and backward, and then all at once darts right to the bottom of the vagina for the ejaculation.

El deukkak (the striker) – Thus called because on arriving at the entrance of the vulva it gives a slight knock. If the vulva opens the door, it enters; if there is no response it begins to knock again, and does not cease until it is admitted. The parasite who wants to get into the house of a rich man to be present at a feast does the same: he knocks at the door; and

if it is opened, he walks in; but if there is no response to his knock, he repeats it again and again until the door is opened. And similarly the deukkak with the door of the vulva.

By "knocking at the door" is meant the friction of the member against the entrance of the vulva until the latter becomes moist. The appearance of this moisture is the phenomenon alluded to by the expression "opening the door."

El aouame (the swimmer) – Because when it enters the vulva it does not remain in one favorite place, but, on the contrary, turns to the right, to the left, goes forward, draws back, and then moves like a simmer in the middle among its own sperm and the fluid furnished by the vulva, as if in fear of drowning and trying to save itself.

El dekhal (the housebreaker) – Merits that name because on coming to the door of the vulva this one asks, "What do you want?" "I want to come in!" Impossible! I cannot take you in on account of your size." Then the member insists that the other one should only receive its head, promising not to come in entirely; it then approaches, rubs its head twice or thrice between the vulva's lips, till

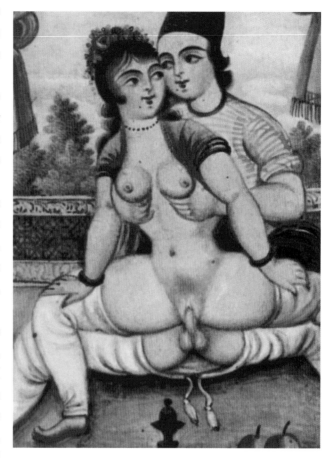

they get humid and thus lubricated, then introduced first its head, and after, with one push, plunges in up to the testicles.

El aouar (the one-eyed) – Because it has but one eye, which eye is not like other eyes, and does not see clearly.

El fortass (the bald one) – Because there is no hair on its head, which makes it look bald.

Abou aine (he with one eye) – It has received this name because it has one eye which presents the peculiarity of being without pupil and eyelashes.

El atsar (the stumbler) – It is called so because if it wants to penetrate into the vulva but does not see the door, it beats about above and below, and thus continues to stumble as over stones in the road, until the lips of the vulva get humid, when it manages to get inside. The vulva then says, "What has happened to you that made you stumble about so?" The members answers, "O my love, it was a stone lying in the road."

El dommar (the odd-headed) – Because its head is different from all other heads.

Abou rokba (the one with a neck) – That is the being with a short neck, a well-developed throat, thick at the end, and a bald head, and who moreover, has coarse and bristly hair from the navel to the pubis.

Abou quetaia (the hairy one; who has a forest of hair) – This name is given to it when the hair is abundant about it.

El besiss (the impudent one) – It has received this name because from the moment that it gets stiff and long it does not care for anybody, lifts impudently the clothing of its master by raising its head fiercely, and makes him ashamed while itself feels no shame. It acts in the same unabashed way with women, turning up their clothes and laying bare their thighs. Its master may blush at this conduct, but as to itself its stiffness and determination to plunge into a vulva only increase.

El mostahi (the shame-faced one) – This sort of member which is met with sometimes, is capable of feeling ashamed and timid when facing a vulva which it does not know, and it is only after a little time that it gets bolder and stiffens. Sometimes it is even so much troubled that it remains incompetent for the coitus, which happens in particular when a stranger is present, in which case it becomes quite incapable of moving.

"When drew she near to bid adieu with heart unstrung,
While care and longing on that day her bosom wrung;
Wet pearls she wept and mine like red carnelians rolled
And, joined in sad rivière, around her neck they hung."

The Arabian Nights

El bekkai (the weeper) – So called on account of the many tears it shed; as soon as it gets in erection, it weeps; when it sees a pretty face, it weeps; handling a woman, it weeps. It goes even so far as to weep tears sacred to memory.

El hezzas (the rummager) – It is named thus because as soon as it penetrates into the vulva it begins to rummage about vigorously, until it has appeased its passion.

El lezzas (the unionist) – Received that name because as soon as it is in the vulva it pushes and works till fur meets fur, and even makes efforts to force the testicles into it.

Abou laaba (the expectorant) – Has received this name because when coming near a vulva, or when it sees one, or even when merely thinking of it, or when its master touches a woman or plays with her or kisses her, its saliva begins to move and it has tears in its eye; this saliva is particularly abundant when it has been for some time out of work, and it will even wet then his master's dress. This member is very common, and there are but few people who are not furnished with it.

The liquid it sheds is cited by lawyers under the name of medi. Its prodcutin is the result of toyings and of lascivious thoughts. With some people it is so abundant as to fill the vulva, so that they may erroneously believe that it comes from the woman.

El fattache (the searcher) – From its habit, when in the vulva, of turning in every direction as if in search of something; and that something is the matrix. It will know no rest until it ha found it.

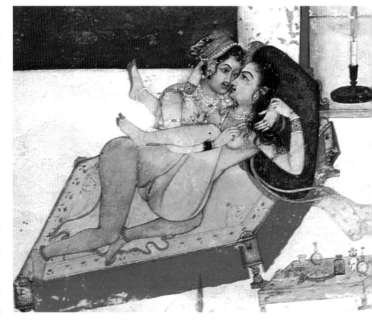

El hakkah (the rubber) – It has got this name because it will not enter the vagina until it has rubbed its head against the entrance and the lower part of the belly. It is frequently mistaken for the next one.

El mourekhi (the flabby one) – This one can never get in because it is too soft, and it is therefore content to rub its head against the entrance to the vulva until it ejaculates. It gives no pleasure to woman, but only inflames her passion without being able to satisfy it, and makes her cross and irritable.

El motela (the ransacker) – So named because it penetrates into the unusual places, makes itself well-acquainted with the state of vulvas, and can distinguish their qualities and faults.

El mokcheuf (the discoverer) – Has been thus denominated because in getting up and raising its head, it raises the vestments which hide it, and uncovers its master's nudities, and because it is also not afraid to lay bare the vulvas which it does not yet know, and to lift up the clothes which cover them without shame. It is not accessible to any sense of bashfulness, cares for nothing and respects nothing. Nothing which concerns the coitus is strange to it; it has a profound knowledge of the state of humidity, freshness, dryness, rightness or warmth of vulvas, which it explores assiduously.

There are, in fact, certain vulvas of an exquisite exterior, plump and fine outside, whose insides leave much to wish for, and they give no pleasure, owning to their being not warm but very humid, and having other similar faults. It is for this reason that the mokcheuf tries to find out about things concerning the coitus, and has received this name.

These are the principal names that have been given to the virile member according to its qualities. Those who think that the number of these names is not exhaustive can look for more; but I think I have given a nomenclature long enough to satisfy my readers.

The Perfumed Garden of the Sheikh Nefzaoui

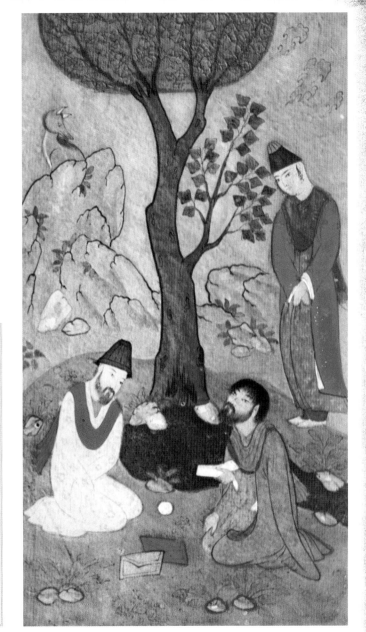

Visit thy lover, spurn what envy told;
No envious churl [ill-bred fellow] shall smile on love ensoul'd
Merciful Allah made no fairer sight
Than coupled lovers single couch doth hold;
Breast pressing breast and robed in joys their own,
With pillowed forearms cast in finest mould;
And when heart speaks to heart with tongue of love,
Folk who would part them hammer steel ice-cold:
If a fair friend thou find who cleaves [clings] to thee,
Live for that friend, that friend in heart enfold.
O ye who blame for love us lover kind
Say, can ye minister to diseased mind?

The Arabian Nights

Chapter 9

The Sundry Names Given to the Sexual Organs of Women

El feurdj, the slit

El keuss, the vulva

El kelmoune, the voluptuous

El ass, the primitive

El zerzour, the starling

El cheukk, the chin

Abou tertour, the one with a cres

Abou khochime, the one with a little nose

El gueunfond, the hedgehog

El sakouti, the silent one

El deukkak, the crusher

El tseguil, the importunate

El taleb, the yearning one

El hacene, the beautiful

El neuffakh, the one that swells

Abou djebaha, the one with a projection

El ouasa, the vast one

El aride, the large one

El harr, the hot one

Abou belaoum, the glutton

El mokaour, the bottomless

Abou cheufrine, the two-lipped

Abou aungra, the humpbacked

El rorbal, the sieve

El hazzaz, the restless

El lezzaz, the unionist

El moudd, the accommodating

El moudine, the assistant

El meusboul, the long one

El molki, the duellist

El harrab, the fugitive

El sabeur, the resigned

El mouseuffah, the barred one

El mezour, the deep one

El addad, the biter

El menssass, the sucker

El zeunbur, the wasp

El ladid, the delicious one

As regards the vulva called el feurdj, the slit, it has this name because it opens and shuts again when hotly yearning for coitus, like the one of a mare in heat at the approach of the stallion. This work, however, is applied indiscriminately to the natural parts of men and women, for God the Supreme has used this expression in the Koran, chap. Xxxiii. V. 35, "El hafidine feuroudjahoum ou el hafidate." The proper meaning of feurdj is slit, opening, passage; people say, "I have found a feurdj in the mountains," viz., a passage; there is then a soukoune upon the ra and fatcha upon the djine, and in this sense it means also the natural parts of woman. But if the ra is marked with a fatcha it signifies deliverance from misfortunes.

The person who dreams of having seen the vulva, feurdj, of a woman will know that "if he is in trouble God will free him of it; if he is in a perplexity he will soon get out of it; and lastly if he is in poverty he will soon become wealthy, because feurdja, by transposing the vowels, will mean the deliverance from evil. By analogy, if he wants a thing he will get it; if he has bets, they will be paid."

It is considered more lucky to dream of the vulva as open. But if the one seen belongs to a young virgin it indicates that the door of consolation will remain closed, and the thing which I desired is not obtainable. It is a proved fact that the man who sees in his dream the vulva of a virgin that has never been touched will certainly be involved in difficulties, and will not be lucky in his affairs. But if the vulva is open so that he can look well into it, or even if it is hidden but he is free to enter it, he will bring the most difficult tasks to a successful end after having first failed in the, and this after a short delay, by the help of a person whom he never thought of.

He who has seen in his dream a man busy upon a young girl, and when the same is getting off her has managed to see at that moment her vulva, will bring his business to a happy end, after having first failed to do so, by the help of the man he has seen. If it is himself who did the girl's business, and he has seen her vulva, he will succeed by his own exertions to realize the most difficult problems, and be successful in every respect. Generally speaking, to see the vulva in dreams is a good sign; so it is good augury to dream of coition, and he who sees himself in the act, and finishing with the ejaculation, will meet success in all his affairs. But it is not the same with the man who merely begins coition and not finish it. He, on the contrary, will be unlucky in every enterprise.

It is supposed that the man who dreams of being busy with a woman will afterwards obtain from her what he wants.

The man who dreams of cohabitating with women with whom to have sexual intercourse is forbidden by religious, as for instance his mother, sister, etc. (maharine), must consider this as a presage that he will go to sacred places (moharreme); and, perhaps, even journey to the holy house of God, and look there upon the grave of the Prophet.

As regards the virile member, it has been previously mentioned that to dream of accident occurring to that organ means the loss of all remembrance and the extinction of the race.

The sight of a pair of pantaloons (seronal) prognosticates the appointment to a post (oulaia) by reason of the analogy of the letters composing the word seronal with those forming by transposition the two words sir, go and auali, named: "Go to the post for which you are named." It is related that a man who had dreamed that the Emir had given him a pair of pantaloons became Cadi. Dreaming of pantaloons is also a sign of protection for the natural parts, and foretells success in business.

The almond (louze), a word composed of the same letters as zal, to cease, seen in a dream by a man in trouble means that he will be liberated from it; to a man who is ill, that he will be cured; in short that all misfortunes will give way. Somebody having dreamed that he was eating almonds, asked a wise man the meaning of it; he received the answer, that by reason of the analogy of the letters in louze and zal, the ills that beset him would disappear; and the event justified the explanation.

The sight of a molar tooth (deurss) in a dream indicates enmity. The man, therefore, who has seen his tooth drop out may be sure that his enemy is dead. This arises from the word deurss, signifying both an enemy and a molar, and one can say at the same time, it is my tooth and it is my enemy.

The wondow (taga) and the shoe (medassa) reminds you of women. The vulva resembles in fact, when invaded by the verge, a window with a man putting his head in to look about, or a shoe that is being put on. Consequently, he who sees himself in dreaming in the act of going in at a window, or putting on a shoe, has the certainty of getting possession of a young woman or a virgin, if the window is newly built, or the shoe new and in good condition; but that woman will be old according to the state of the window or shoe.

The loss of a shoe foretells to a man the loss of his wife.

To dream of something folded together, and which gets open, predicts that a secret will be divulged and made public. The same remaining folded up indicates, on the other hand, that the secret will be kept.

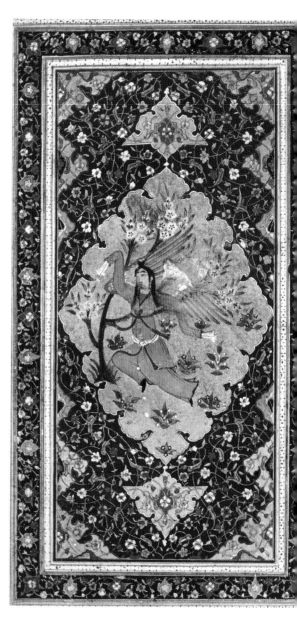

If you dream of reading a letter you will know that you will have news, which will be, according to the nature of the contents of the letter, good or bad.

The man who drams of passages in the Koran or the Traditions, Hadits, will from the subjects treated therein draw his conclusions. For instance, the passage, "He will grant you the help of God and immediate victory," will signify to him victory and triumph. "Certainly he (God) has the decision in his hands, "Heaven will open and offer its numerous portals, and other similar passages, indicate success.

A passage treating of punishments prognosticates punishment; from those treating of benefits a lucky event may be concluded. Such is the passage in the Koran, which says: "He who forgives sins is terrible in his inflictions."

Dreams about poetry and songs contain their explanation in the contents of the objects of the dream.

He who dreams of horses, mules, or asses may hope for good, for the Prophet (God's salutation and goodness be with him!) has said, "Men's fortunes are attached to the forelocks of their horses till the day of resurrection!" and it is written I the Koran, "God the Highest has thus willed it that they serve you for mounts and for state."

The correctness of these prognostications is not subject to any doubt.

He who dreams of seeing himself mounted upon an ass as a courier, and arriving at his destination, will be lucky in all things; but he would tumbles off the ass on his way is advised that he will be subject to accidents and misfortunes.

The fall of the turban from the head predicts ignominy, the turban being the Arab's crown.

If you see yourself in a dream with naked feet it means a loss; and the bare head has the same significance.

By transposing the letters other analogies may be arrived at.

These explanations are not here in their place; but I have been induced to give them in their chapter on account of the use to which they may be put. Persons who would wish to know more on this subject have only to consult the treatise of Ben Sirine. I now return to the names given to the sexual part of woman.

El keuss (the vulva) – This word serves as the name of a young woman's vulva in particular. Such a vulva is very plump and round in every direction, with long lips, grand slit, the edges well-divided and symmetrical and rounded; it is soft, seductive, perfect throughout. It is the most pleasant and no doubt the best of all the different sorts. May God grant us the possession of such a vulva! Amen. It is warm, tight, and dry; so much so that one might expect to see fire burst from it. Its form is graceful, its odor pleasant; the whiteness of its outside sets off its carmine-red middle. There is no imperfection about it.

El kelmoune (the voluptuous) – The name given to the vulva of a young virgin.

El ass (the primitive) – This is a name applicable to every kind of vulva.

El zerzour (the starling) – The vulva of a very young girl, or, as other pretend, of a brunette.

El cheukk (the chink) – The vulva of a bony, lean woman. It is like a chink in a wall, with not a vestige of flesh. May God keep us from it!

Abou tertour (the crested one) – It is the name given to a vulva furnished with a red comb, like that of a cokc, which rises at the moment of enjoyment.

Abou khochime (the snub-nose) – It is a vulva with thin lips and a small tongue.

El gueunfond (the hedgehog) – The vulva of the old, decrepit woman, dried up with age and with bristly hair.

El sakouti (the silent one) – This name has been given to the vulva that is noiseless. The member may enter it a hundred times a day but it will not say a word, and will be content to look on without a murmur.

El deukkak (the crusher) – So called from its crusihing movements upon the member. It generally begins to push the

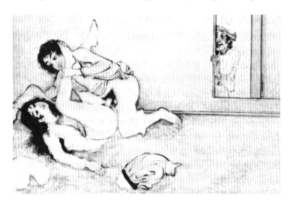

The Savage

Ameenah was a stunning black slave with a gorgeous body and fine face, and she moved with the grace of a dangerous wild animal. Holding on to me for dear life, she would reach orgasm frequently and wildly, emitting a low-pitched but otherwise piercing shriek. When this happened, she would spread her legs even wider, but she would stop moving. At that point, I could feel the rapid contractions of her vagina, accompanied by her sobbing gasps. With back arched, she would press her breasts against me. This was the signal for me to take one of them in my mouth and suck hard. She would scream repeatedly and tremble like a leaf in a gale. I once made the mistake of trying to kiss her when she was in that state, but she bit me savagely, and I still have the scar on my lips.

She enjoyed fifteen-second orgasms, after which she calmed down completely for a short while – until her lust was rekindled and she began to move again.

The Fountains of Pleasure

member, directly it enters, to the right and to the left, and to grip it with the matrix, and would, if it could, absorb also the two testicles.

El tseguil (the importunate) – This is the vulva which is never tired of taking in the member. This latter might pass a hundred nights with it, and walk a hundred times every night, still that vulva would not be sated – nay, it would want still more, and would not allow the member to come out again at all, if it was possible. With such a vulva the parts are exchanged; the vulva is the pursuer, the member the pursued. Luckily it is a rarity, and only found in a small number of women, who are wild with passion, all on fire, and in flame.

El taleb (the yearning one) – This vagina is met with in a few women only. With some it is natural; with others it becomes what it is by long abstinence. It is burning for a member, and, having got one in its embrace, it refuses to part with it until its fire is completely extinguished.

El hacene (the beautiful) – This is the vulva which is white, plump, in form vaulted like a dome, firm, and without any deformity. You cannot take your eyes off it, and to look at it changes a feeble erection in a strong one.

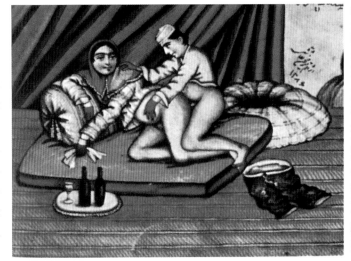

El neuffakh (the swelling one) – So called because a torpid member coming near it, and rubbing its head against it a few times, at once swells and stands upright. To the woman who has such a one it procures excessive pleasure, for, at the moment of the crisis, it opens and shuts convulsively, like the vulva of a mare.

Abou djebaha (one with a projection) – Some women have this sort of vulva, which is very large, with a pubis prominent like a projecting, fleshy forehead.

El ouasa (the vast one) – A vulva surrounded by a very large pubis. Women of that build are said to be of large vagina, because, although on the approach of the member it appears firm and impenetrable to such a degree that not even a meroud seems likely to be passed in, as soon as it feels the friction of the glans against its center it opens wide at once.

El aride (the large one) – This is the vulva which is as wide as it is long; that is to say, fully developed all around, from side to side, and from the pubis to the perineum. It is the most beautiful to look upon. As the poet said:

> It has the splendid whiteness of a forehead,
> In its dimensions it is like the moon,
> The fire that radiates from it is like the sun's,
> And seems to burn the member which approaches;
> Unless first moistened with saliva the member cannot enter,
> The odor it emits is full of charms.

It is also said that this name applies to the vagina of women who are plump and fat. When such a one crosses her thighs one over the other, the vulva stands out like the head of a calf. If she lays it bare it resembles a saa for corn placed between her thighs; and, if she walks, it is apparent under her clothes by its wavy movement at each step. May God, in his goodness and generosity, let us enjoy such a vagina! It is of all the most pleasing, the most celebrated, the most wished for.

Abou belaoum (the glutton) – The vulva with a vast capacity for swelling. If such a vulva has not been able to get coitus for some time it fairly engulfs the member that then comes near it, without leaving any trace of it outside, like as a man who is famished flings himself upon viands that are offered to him, and would swallow them without mastication.

El mokaour (the bottomless) – This is the vagina of the indefinite length, having, in consequence, the matrix lying very far back. It requires a member of the largest dimensions; any other could not succeed in rousing its amorous sensibilities.

Abou cheufrine (the two-lipped) – This name is given to the amply developed vagina of an excessively stout woman. Also to the vagina the lips of which having become flaccid, owing to weakness, are long and pendulous.

Abou aungra (the humpbacked) – This vulva has the mount of Venus prominent and hard, standing out like the hump on the back of the camel, and reaching down between the thighs like the head of a calf. May God let us enjoy such a vulva! Amen!

El rorbal (the sieve) – This vulva on receiving a member seems to sift it all over, below, right and left, fore and aft, until the moment of pleasure arrives.

El hazzaz (the restless) – When this vagina has received the member it begins to move violently and without interruption until the member touches the matrix, and then knows no repose till it has hastened on the enjoyment and finished its work.

El lezzaz (the unionist) – This vagina which, having taken in the member, clings to it and pushes itself forward upon it so closely that, if the thing were possible, it would enfold the two testicles.

El moudd (the accommodating) – This name is applied to the vagina of a woman who has felt for a long time an ardent wish for coition. In rapture with the member it sees, it is glad to second its movements of come and go; it offers its matrix to the member by pressing it forward within reach, which is, after all, the best gift it can offer. Whatever place inside of it the member wants to explore, this vulva will make him welcome to, gracefully according to its wish; there is no corner it will not help the member to reach.

El moudine (the assistant) – This vulva is thus named because it assists the member to go in and out, to go up and down, in short, in all its movements, in such a way that if it desires to do a thing, to enter or to retire, to move about, etc., the vulva hastens to give it all facilities, and answers to its appeal. By this aid the ejaculation is facilitated, and the enjoyment heightened.

El meusboul (the long one) – This name applies only to some vulvas; everyone knows that vulvas are far from being all of the same conformation and aspect. This vulva extends from the pubis to the anus. It lengthens out when the woman is lying down or standing, and contracts when she is sitting, differing in this respect from the vulva of a round shape. It looks like a splendid cucumber lying between the thighs. With some women it shows projecting under light clothing, or when they are bending back.

El molki (the duelist) – This is the vulva which, on the introduction of a member, executes the movement of coming and going, pushes itself upon it for fear of its retiring before the pleasure arrives. There is no enjoyment for it but the shock given to its matrix by the member, and it is for this that it projects its matrix to girfp and such the member's gland when the ejaculation takes place. Certain vulvas, wild with desire and lust, be it natural or a consequence of long abstention, throw themselves upon the approaching ember, opening the mouth like a famished infant to whom the mother offers the breast. In the same way this vulva advances and retires upon the member to bring it face to face with the matrix, as if in fear that, unaided, it could not find the same.

The vulva and the member resemble thus two skillful duelists, each time that one of them rushes its antagonist, the latter opposes it shield to parry the blow and repulse the assault. The member represents the sword, and the matrix the shield. The one who first ejaculates and sperm is vanquished; while the one who is slowest is the victor; and, assuredly, it is a fine fight! I should like thus to fight without stopping to the day of my death.

As the poet says:

I have let them see the effect of a subtle shadow,
Spinning like an every busy spider
They said to me, "How long will you go on?"
I answered the, "I will work till I am dead."

El harrab (the fugitive) – The vagina which, being very tight and short, is hurt by the penetration of a very large and soft member; it tries to escape to the right and left. It is thus, people say, like the vagina of most virgins, which, not yet having made the acquaintance of the member and fearful of its approach, tries to get out of its way when it glides in between the thighs and wants to be admitted.

El sabeur (the resigned) – This is the vulva which, having admitted the member, submits pateitnly to all its whims, and movements. It is also said that this vulva is strong enough to suffer resignedly the most violent and prolonged coitus. If it were assaulted a hundred times it would not be vexed or annoyed; and instead of venting reproaches, it would give thanks to God. It will show the same patience if it has to do with several members who visit it successively.

This kind of vagina is found in women of a glowing terparament. If they only knew how to do it, they would not allow the man to dismount, nor his member to retire for a single moment.

El mouseuffah (the barred one) – This kind of vagina is not often met with. The defect which distinguished it is sometimes natural, sometimes it is the result of an unskillfully executive operation of circumcision upon the woman. It can happen that the operator makes a false move with his instrument and injures the two lips, or even only one of them. In healing there forms a thick scar, which bars the passage, and in order to make the vagina accessible to the member, a surgical operation and the use of the bistouri will have to be resorted to.

El addad (the biter) – The vulva which, when the member has got into it and is burning with passion, opens and shuts again upon the same fiercely. It is chiefly when the ejaculation is coming that the man feels the head of his member bitten by the mouth of the matrix. And certainly there is an attractive power in the same when it clings, yearning for sperm, to the gland, and draws it in as far as it can. If God in his power has decreed that the woman shall become pregnant the sperm gets concentrated in the matrix, where it is gradually vivified; but if, on the contrary, God does not permit the conception, the matrix expels the seed, which then runs over the vagina.

El menssass (the sucker) – This is a vagina which in its amorous heat in consequence of voluptuous toyings, or of long abstinence, begins to suck the member which as entered it so forcibly as to deprive it of all the its perm, dealing with it as a child drawing on the breast of the mother.

The poets have described it in the following verse:

> *She – the woman – shows in turning up her robe*
> *An object – the vulva – developed full and round,*
> *In semblance like a cup turned upside down.*
> *In placing thereupon your hand, you seem to feel*
> *A well-formed bosom, springy, firm, and full.*
> *In boring your lance it gets well bitten,*
> *And drawn in by a suction, as the breast is by a child,*
> *You'll find it flaming hot as any furnace.*

Another poet (may God grant all his wishes in Paradies!) has composed on the same theme the following lines:

> *Like to a man extended on his chest, she – the vulva – fills the hand*
> *Which has to be well stretched to cover it.*
> *The place it occupies is standing forth*
> *Like an unopened bud of the blossom of a plum tree.*
> *Assuredly the smoothness of its skin*
> *Is like the beardless cheek of adolescence;*
> *Its conduit is but narrow,*

The entrance to it is not easy,

And he who essays to get in

Feels as though he was butting against a coat of mail,

And at the introduction it emits a sound

Like to the tearing of a woven stuff.

The member having filled its cavity,

Receives the lively welcome of a bit,

Such as the nipple of the nurse receives

When placed between the nursling's lips for suction.

Its lips are burning,

Like a fire that is lighted,

And how sweet it is, this fire!

How delicious for me.

El zeunbur (the wasp) – This kind of vulva is known by the strength and roughness of its fur. When the member approaches and tries to enter it gets stung by the hairs as if by a wasp.

El harr (the hot one) – This is one of the most praiseworthy vulvas. Warm is in fact very much esteemed in a vulva, and it may be said that the intensity of the enjoyment afforded by it is in proportion to the heat it develops.

Poets have praised it in the following verses:

The vulva possesses an intrinsic heat;

Shut in a solid heart (interior) and pent up breast (matrix).

Its fire communicates itself to him that enters it;

It equals in intensity the fire of love.

She is as tight as a well-fitting shoe,

Smaller than the circle of the apple of the eye.

El ladid (the delicious one) – It has the reputation of procuring an unexampled pleasure, comparable only to the one felt by the beasts and birds of prey, and for which they fight sanguinary combats. And if such effects are produced upon animals, what must they be for man? And so it is that all wars spring from the search for the voluptuous pleasure which the vagina procures, and which is the highest fortune of this world; it is a part of the delights of paradise awarded to us by God as a foretaste of what is waiting for us, namely, delights a thousand times superior, and above which only the sight of the Benevolent (God) is to be placed.

More names might certainly be found applicable to the sexual organs of woman, but the number of those mentioned above appears to me ample. The principal object of this work is to collect together all the remarkable and attractive matters concerning coitus, so that he who is in trouble may find consolation in it, and the man to whom erection offers difficulties may be able to look into it for a remedy against his weakness. Wise physicians have written that people whose members have lost their strength, and are afflicted with impotence, should assiduously read books treating of coition, and study carefully the different kind of lovemaking, in order to recover their former vigor. A coition. As it is not always everywhere possible to see animals while in the act of copulation, books on the subject of generation are indispensable. In every country, large or small, both the rich and poor have a taste for this sort of book, which may be compared to the stone of philosophy transforming common metals into gold

It is related (and God penetrates the most obscure matters, and is most wise!) that once upon a time, before the reign of the great Caliph Haroun er Rachid, there lived a buffoon, who was the amusement of women, old people and children. His name was Djoaidi. Many women granted him their favors freely, and he was much-liked and well received by all. By princes, viziers and caids he was likewise very well treated; in general all the world pampered him; at that time, indeed, any man that was a buffoon enjoyed the greatest consideration, for which reason the poet has said:

> Oh, Time! Of all the dwellers here below
> You only elevate buffoons or fools,
> Or him whose mother was a prostitute,
> Or him whose anus as an inkstand serves,
> Or him who from his youth has been a pander;
> Who has no other work but to bring the two sexes together.

The History of Djoaidi and Fadahat el Djemal

I was in love with a woman who was all grace and perfection, beautiful of shape, and gifted with all imaginable charms. Her cheeks were like roses, her forehead lily white, her lips like coral; she had teeth like pearls, and breasts like pomegranates. Her mouth opened round like a ring; her tongue seemed to be incrusted with precious gems; her eyes black and finely slit, had the languor of slumber, and her voice the sweetness of sugar. With her form pleasantly filled out, her flesh was mellow like fresh butter, and pure as the diamond.

As to her vulva, it was white, prominent, round as an arch; the center of it was red, and breathed fire, without a trace of humidity; for, sweet to the touch, it was quite dry. When she walked it showed in relief like a dome or an inverted cup. In reclining it was visible between her thighs, looking like a kid couched on a hillock.

This woman was my neighbor. All the others played and laughed with me, jested with me, and met my suggestions with great pleasure. I reveled in their kisses, their close embraces and nibbling, and in sucking their lips, breasts, and necks. I had coition with all of them, except my neighbor, and it was exactly her I wanted to possess in preference to all the rest; but instead of being kind to me, she avoided me rather. When I contrived to take her aside to trifle with her and try to rouse her gaiety, and spoke to her of my desires, she recited to me the following verses, the sense of which was a mystery to me:

Among the mountain tops I saw a tent placed firmly,
Apparent to all eyes high up in mid-air.
But, oh! The pole that held it up was gone.
And like a vase without a handle it remained,
With all its cords undone, its center sinking in,
Forming a hollow like that of a kettle.

Every time I told her of my passion, she answered me with these verses, which to me were void of meaning, and to which I could make no reply, which, however, only excited my love all the more. I therefore inquired of all those I knew – among wise men, philosophers, and savants – the meaning, but not one of them could solve the riddle for me, so as to satisfy my heat and appease my passion.

Nevertheless I continued my investigations, until at last I heard of a savant name Abou Nouass, who lived in a far-off country, and who, I was told, was the only man capable of solving the enigma. I betook to him, apprised him of the distress I had with the woman, and recited to him the above-mentioned verses.

About Nouass said to me, "This woman loves you to the exclusion of every other man. She is very corpulent and plump." I answered, "It is exactly as you say. You have given her likeness as if she were before you, excepting what you say in respect of her love for me, for until now, she has never given me any proof of it."

"She has no husband."

"This is so," I said.

Then he added, "I have reason to believe that your member is of small dimensions, and such a member cannot give her pleasure nor quench her fire; for what she wants is a lover with a member like this!" When I had reassured him on that point, affirming that my member, which began to rise at the expression of his doubtings, was full-sized, he told me that in that case all difficulties would disappear, and explained to me the sense of the verses as follows:

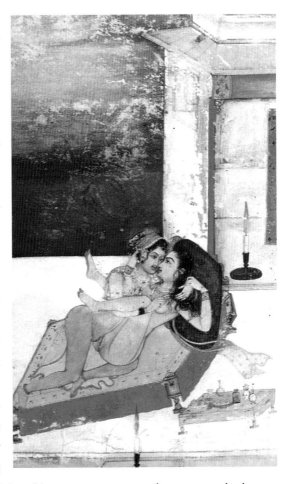

The tent, firmly planted, represents the vulva of grand dimension and placed well forward, the mountains, between which it rises, are the thighs. The stake which supported its center and has been torn up means that she has no husband, comparing the stake or pole that supports the tent to the virile member holding up the lips of the vulva. She is like a vase without a handle; this means if the pail is without a handle to hang it up by it is good for nothing, the pail representing the vulva, and the handle the verge. The cords are undone and its center is sinking in; that is to say, as the tent without a supporting pole caves in at the center, inferior in this respect to the vault which remains upright without support, so can the woman who has no husband not enjoy complete happiness. From the words, It forms a hollow like that of a kettle, you may judge how lascivious God has made that woman in her comparisons; she likens her vulva to a kettle, which serves to prepare the

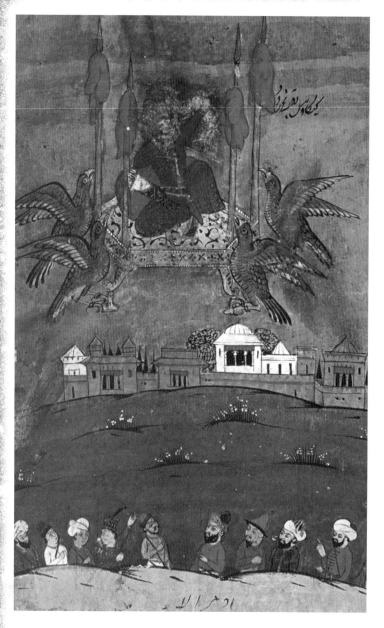

tserid. Listen; if the tserid is placed in the kettle, to turn out well it must be stirred by means of a medeleuk, long and solid, while the kettle is steadied by the feet and hands. Only in that way can it be properly prepared. It cannot e done with a small spoon; the cook would burn her hands, owing to the shortness of the handle, and the dish would not be well-prepared. This is the symbol of this woman's nature, O Djoaidi. If your member has not the dimensions of a respectable medeleuk, serviceable for the good preparation of the tserid, it will not give her satisfaction, and moreover, if you do not hold her close to your chest, enlacing her with your hands and feet, it is useless to solicit her favors; finally if you let her consume herself by her own fire, like the bottom of the kettle which gets burned if the medeleuk is not stirred upon it, you will not gratify her desire by the result.

"You see now what prevented her from acceding to your wishes; she was afraid that you would not be able to quench her flame after having fanned it.

"But what is the name of this woman, O Djoaidi?"

"Fadehat el Djemal" (the sunrise of beauty), I replied.

"Return to her," said the sage, "and take her these verses, and your affair will come to a happy issue, please God! You will then come back to me, and inform me of what will have come to pass between you two."

I gave my promise, and Abou Nouass recited to me the following lines:

Have patience now, O Fadehat el Djemal,
I understand your words, and all shall see how I obey them.
O you! Beloved and cherished by whoever
Can revel in your charms and glory in them!
O apple of my eye! You thought I was embarrassed
About the answer which I had to give you.
Yes, certainly! It was the love I bore you
Made me look foolish in the eyes of all you know.
They thought I was possessed of a demon;
Called me a Merry Andrew and buffoon.
For God! What a buffoonery I've got,
Should it be that
No other member is like mine? Here! See it, measure it!
What woman tastes it falls in love with me,
In violent love. It is a well-known fact
That you from far may see it like a column.
If it erects itself it lifts my robe and shames me.
Now take it kindly, put it in your tent,
Which is between the well-known mountains placed.
It will be quite at home there, you will find it
Not softening while inside, but sticking like a nail;
Take it to form a handle to your vase.
Come and examine it, and notice well

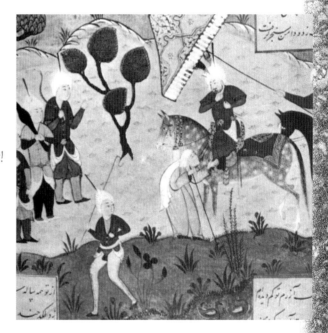

How vigorous it is and long in its erection!
If you but want a proper medeleuk,
A medeleuk to use between your thighs,
Take this to stir the center of your kettle.
It will do good to you, O mistress mine!
Your kettle be it plated will be satisfied!

Having learned these verses by heart, I took my leave of Abou Nouass and returned to Fadehat el Djemal. She was, as usual, alone. I gave a slight knock at her door; she came out at once, beautiful as the rising sun, and coming up to me, she said,

"Oh! Enemy of God, what business has brought you here to me at this time?" I answered her, "O my mistress! A business of great importance."

"Explain yourself, and I will see whether I can help you," she said.

"I shall not speak to you about it until the door is locked," I answered.

"Your boldness today is very great," she said.

And I, "True, O my mistress! Boldness is one of my qualities."

She then addressed me thus, "O enemy of yourself! O you most miserable of your race! If I were to lock the door, and you have nothing wherewith to satisfy my desires, what should I do with you? Face of a Jew!"

"You will let me share your couch, and grant me your favors."

She began to laugh; and after we had entered the house, she told a slave to lock the house door. As usual, I asked her to respond to my proposals; she then recited to me again the above-mentioned verses. When she had finished I began to recite to her those which Abou Nouass had taught me.

As I proceeded I saw her more and more moved, I observed her giving way to yawns, to stretch herself, to sigh. I knew now I should arrive at the desired result. When I had finished, my member was in such a state of erection that it became like a pillar, still lengthening. When Fadehat el Djemal saw it in that condition she precipitated herself upon it, took it into her hands, and drew it towards her thighs. I then said, "O apple of my eyes! This may not be done here, let us go into your chamber."

She replied, "Leave me alone, O son of a debauched woman! Before God! I am losing my senses in seeing your member getting longer and longer, and lifting your robe. Oh, what a member! I never saw a finer one! Let it penetrate into this delicious, plump vulva, which maddens all who hear it described; for the sake of which so many have died of love; and which your superiors and masters themselves have not been able to get possession."

I repeated, "I shall not do it anywhere else than in your chamber."

She answered, "If you do not enter this minute this tender vulva, I shall die."

As I still insisted upon repairing to her room, she cried, "No, it is quite impossible; I cannot wait so long!"

I saw in fact her lips tremble, her eyes filling with tears. A general tremor ram over her , she changed color, and laid herself down upon her back, baring her thighs, the whiteness of which made her flesh appear like crystal tinged with carmine.

Then I examined her vulva – a white cupola with a purple center, soft and charming. It opened like that of a mare on the approach of a stallion.

At that moment she seized my member and kissed it, saying, By the religion of my father! It must penetrate into my vulva! And drawing nearer to me she pulled it towards her vagina.

I now hesitated no longer to assist her with my member, and placed it against the entrance to her

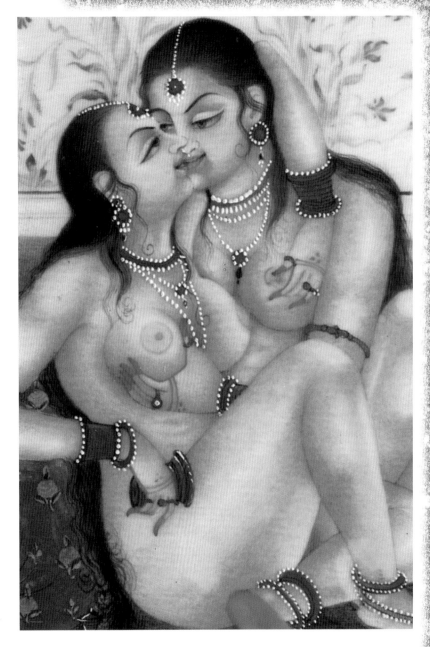

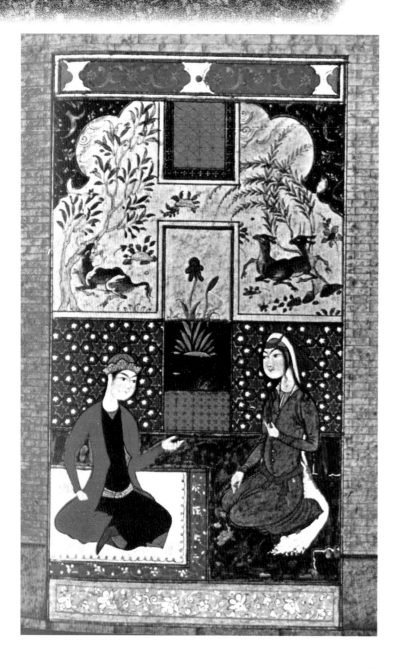

The woman in perpetuum mobile

I married an Egyptian girl called Muneerah when she was fourteen. She had an hourglass figure with a tiny waist and full hips, her shiny black hair hung down her back like a curtain and her skin was golden.

Although she had never been with a man when I married her, she was a quick and talented learner, and applied herself enthusiastically to her training in sexual techniques. She could not stop moving from the second I penetrated her. It was an incredible feeling to have her reach orgasm quickly and frequently, never staying still for a second, and moaning blissfully all the time. Her eyes would stare unseeingly throughout the entire procedure, and her vagina was dripping wet.

Because of the constant stimulation of her squirming movements, I had a hard time holding my own orgasm back. I don't remember every encountering a woman like her.

The Fountains of Pleasure

vulva. As soon as the head of my member touched the lips, the whole body of Fadehat el Djemal trembled with excitement. Sighing and sobbing, she held me pressed to her bosom.

Again I profited by this moment to admire the beauties of her vulva. It was magnificent, its purple center setting off its whiteness all the more. It was round, and without any imperfection; projecting like a splendidly curved dome over her belly. In one word, it was a masterpiece of creation as fine as could be seen. The blessing of God, the best creator, upon it.

And the woman who possessed this wonder had in her time no superior.

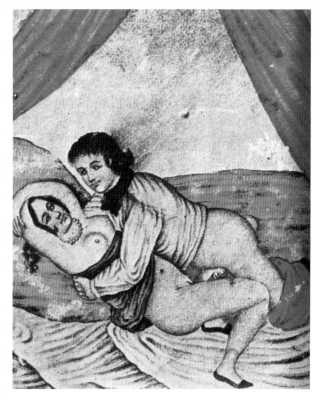

Seeing her then in such transports, trembling like a bird, the throat of which is being cut, I pushed my dart into her. Thinking she might not be able to take in the hole of my member, I had entered cautiously, but she moved her buttocks furiously, saying to me, "This is not enough for my contentment." Making a strong push, I lodged my member completely in her, which made her utter a painful cry, but the moment after she moved with greater fury than before. She cried, "Do not miss the corners, neither high nor low, but above all things do not neglect the center! The center!" she repeated. "If you feel it coming, let it go into my matrix so as to extinguish my fire." Then we moved alternately in and out, which was delicious. Our legs were interlaced, our muscles unbent, and so we went on with kisses and claspings, until the crisis came upon us simultaneously. We then rested and took breath after this mutual conflict.

I wanted to withdraw my member, but she would not consent to his and begged of me not to take it out. I acceded to her wish, but a moment later she took it out herself, dried it, and replaced it in her vulva. We renewed our game, kissing, pressing, and moving in rhythm. After a short time, we rose and entered her chamber, without having this time accomplished the enjoyment. She game me now a piece of an aromatic root, which he recommended me to keep in my mouth, assuring me that as long as I had it there my member would remain on the alert. Then she asked me to lie down, which I did. She mounted upon me, and taking my member into her hands, she made it enter entirely into her vagina. I was astonished at the vigor of her vulva and at the heat emitted from it. The opening of her matrix in particular excited my admiration. I never had any experience like it; it closely clasped my member and pinched gland.

With the exception of Fadehat el Djemal no woman had until then taken in my member to its full length. She was able to do so, I believe, owing to her being very plump and corpulent, and her vulva being large and deep.

Fadehat el Djemal, astride upon me, began to rise and descend; she kept crying out, wept, went slower, then accelerated her movements again, ceased to move altogether; when part of my member became visible she looked at it, then took it out altogether to examine it closely, then plunged it in again until it had appeared completely. So she continued until the enjoyment overcame her again. At last, having dismounted from me, she now laid herself down, and asked me to get on to her. I did so, and she introduced my member entirely into her vulva.

We thus continued our caresses, changing our positions in turns until night came on. I thought it proper to show a wish to go now, but she would not agree to this, and I had to give her my word that I would remain. I said to myself. "This woman will not let me go at any price, but when daylight comes God will advise me." I remained with her, and all night long we kept caressing each other, and took but scanty rest.

I counted that during that day and night, I accomplished twenty-seven times the act of coitus, and I became afraid that I should nevermore be able to leave the house of that woman.

Having at last made good my escape, I went to visit Abou Nouass again, and informed him of all that had happened. He was surprised and stupefied, and his first words were, "O Djoaidi, you can have neither authority nor power over such a woman, and would make you do penance for all the pleasure you have had with other women!"

However, Fadehat el Djemal proposed to me to become her legitimate husband, in order to put a stop to the vexatious rumors that were circulating about her conduct. I, on the other hand, was only on the look out for adultery. Asking the advice of Abou Nouass about it, he told me, "If you marry Fadehat el Djemal you will ruin your health, and God will withdraw his protection from you, and the worst of all will be that she will cuckold you, for she is insatiable with respect to the coitus, and would cover you with shame." And I answered him, "Such is the nature of women; they are insatiable as far as their vulvas are concerned, and so long as their lust is satisfied they do not care whether it be with a buffoon, a Negro, a valet, or even with a man that is despised and reprobated by society."

On this occasion Abou Nouass depicted the character of women in the following verses:

Women are demons, and were born as such;
No one can trust them, as is known to all;
If they love a man, it is only out of caprice;
And he to whom they are most cruel loves them most;
Beings full of treachery and trickery, I aver
The man that loves you truly is a lost man;
He who believes me not can prove my word
By letting woman's love get hold of him for years!
If in your own generous mood you have given them
Your all and everything for years and years,
They will say afterwards, "I swear by God! My eyes
Have never seen a thing he gave me!"
After you have impoverished yourself for their sake,
Their cry from day to day will be forever, "Give!
Give, man. Get up and buy and borrow."
If they cannot profit by you they'll turn against you;
They will tell lies about you and calumniate you.
They do not recoil to use a slave in the master's absence,
If once their passions are aroused, and they play tricks;
Assuredly, if once their vulva is in rut,
They only think of getting some member in erection.
Preserve us, God! From woman's trickery;
And of old women in particular. So be it.

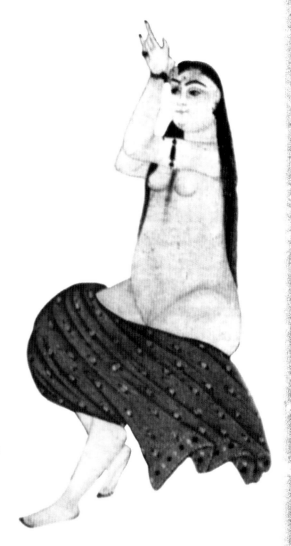

The Perfumed Garden of the Sheikh Nefzaoui

Chapter 10

Concerning the Organs of Generation of animals

Know, O Vizir (God's blessing be with you!), that the sexual organs of the various male animals are not analogous with the different natures of the virile members which I have mentioned.

The verges of animals are classed according to the species to which they belong, and these species are four in number.

1. The verges of animals with hoofs, as the horse, mule, ass, which verges are of large size.

El rermoul, the colossus

El kass, the serpent rolled up

El fellag, the splitter

El zellate, the club

El hearmak, the indomitable

El meunefoukh, the swollen

Abou dommar, the one with a head

Abou beurnita, the one with a hat

El kerukite, the pointed staff

El keuntra, the bridge

El rezama, the mallet

Abou sella, the fighter

2. The verges of animals which have the kind of feet called akhefaf, as, for instance, the camel.

El maloum, the well-known

El tonil, the long one

El cherita, the riband

El mostakime, the firm one

El heurkal, the swinging one

El mokheubbi, the hidden one

El chaaf, the tuft

Tsequil el ifaha, the slow-coach

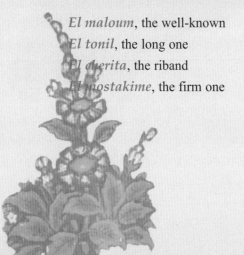

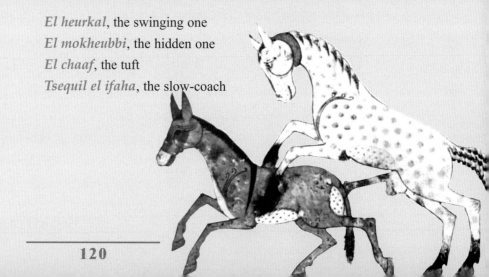

3. The verges of animals with split hooves, like the ox, the sheep, etc.

El aceub, the nerve

El heurbadj, the rod

El sonte, the whip

Requig er ras, the small head

El tonil, the long one

El aicoub, the nervous (for the ram)

4. And lastly, the members of animals with claws, as the lion, fox, dog, and other animals of this species.

El kedib, the verge

El kibouss, the great gland

El metemerole, the one that will lengthen

It is believed that of all the animals of God's creation the lion is the most expert in respect to coition. If he meets the lioness he examines her before copulation. He will know if she has already been covered by a male. When she comes to him he smells at her, and if she has allowed herself to be crossed by a boar he knows it immediately by the odor that animal has left upon her. He then smells her urine, and if the examination proves unfavorable, he gets into a rage, and begins to lash with his tail right and left. Woe to the animal that comes at that time near him; it is certain to be torn to pieces. He then returns to the lioness, who seeing that he knows all, trembles with terror. He smells again at her, utters a roar which makes the mountains shake, and falling upon her, lacerates her back with his claws. He even will go so far as to kill her, and then befoul her body with his urine.

It is said that the lion is the most jealous and most intelligent of all animals. It is also averred that he is generous, and spares him who gets round him by fair words.

A man who on meeting a ion uncovers his sexual parts causes him to take flight.

Whoever pronounces before a lion the name of Daniel (hail be to him!) also sends him flying, because the prophet (hail be to him!) has enjoined this upon the lion in respect to the invocation of his name. Therefore, when this name is pronounced the lion departs without doing any harm. Several cases which prove this fact are cited.

The Perfumed Garden of the Sheikh Nefzaoui

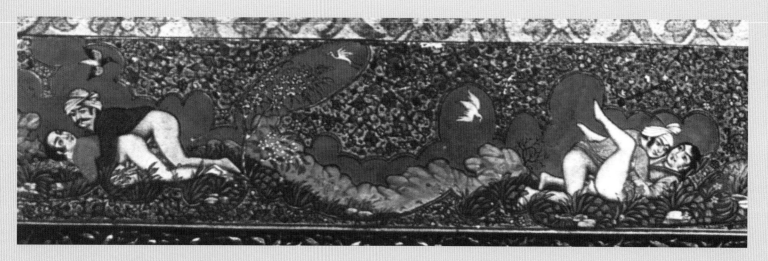

On the Deceits and Treacheries of Women

Know, O Vizir (to whom God be good!), that the stratagems of women are numerous and ingenious. Their tricks will deceive Satan himself, for God the Highest has said (Koran, chapter xii, verse 28, that the deceptive faculties of women are great, and he has likewise said (Koran, chapter vi, verse 38) that the stratagems of Satan are weak. Comparing the word of God as to the ruses of Satan and woman, contained in those two verses, it is easy to see how great these latter ones are.

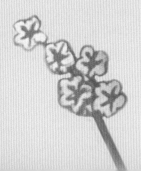

Story of a Deceived Husband being Convicted Himself of Infidelity

It is related that a man fell in love with a woman of great beauty, and possessing all perfections imaginable. He made many advances to her, which were repulsed; then he had endeavored to seduce her by rich presents, which were likewise declined. He lamented, complained, and was prodigal with his money in order to conquer her, but to no purpose, and he grew lean as a specter.

This lasted for some time, when he made the acquaintance of an old woman, whom he took into his confidence, complaining bitterly about it. She said to him, "I shall help you, please God."

Forthwith she made her way to the house of the woman, in order to get an interview with her; but on arriving there the neighbors told her that she could not get in, because the house was guarded by a ferocious bitch, who did not allow anyone to come in or to depart, and in her malignity always flew at the faces of people.

Hearing this, the old woman rejoiced, and said to herself, "I shall succeed, please God." She then went home, and filled a basket with bits of meat. Thus provided, she returned to the woman's house, and went in.

The bit, on seeing her, rose to spring at her; but she produced the basket with its contents, and showed it to her. As soon as the brute saw the viands, it showed its satisfaction by the movements of its tail and nostrils. The old woman putting down the basket before it, spoke to it as follows, "Eat, O my sister. Your absence has been painful to me; I did not know what had become of you, and I have been looking for you a long time. Appease your hunger!

While the animal was eating, and she stroked its back, the mistress of the house came to see who was there, and was not a little surprised to see the bitch, which would never suffer anybody to come near her, so friendly with a strange person. She said, "O old woman, how is it that you know our dog?" The old woman gave no reply, but continued to caress the animal, and utter lamentations.

Then said the mistress of the house to her, "My heart aches to see you thus. Tell me the cause of your sorrow.

"This bitch," said the woman, "was formerly a woman, and my best friend. One fine day she was invited with me to a wedding' she put on her best clothes, and adorned herself with her finest ornaments. We then went together. On our way we were accosted by a man, who at her sight was seized with the most violent love; but she would not listen to him. Then he offered brilliant presents, which she also declined. This man, meeting her some days later, said to her, "Surrender yourself to my passion, or else I shall conjure God to change you into a bitch." She answered, "Conjure as much as you like." The man then called the maledictions of heaven upon that woman, and she was changed into a bitch as you can see here."

At these words the mistress of the house began to cry and lament, saying "O, my mother! I am afraid that I shall meet the same fate as this bitch." Why, what have you done?" said the old woman. The other answered, "There is a man who has loved me since a long time, and I have refused to accede to his desires, nor did I listen to him, though the saliva was dried up in his mouth by his supplications; and in spite of the large expenses he had gone to in order to gain my favor, I have always answered him that I should not consent; and now, O my mother, I am afraid that he might call to God to curse me.

"Tell me how to know this man, " said the old woman, "for fear that you might become like this animal."

"Bur how will you be able to find him, and whom could I send to him?"

The old woman answered, "Me, daughter of mine! I shall render you this service, and find him."

"Make haste, O my mother, and see him before he conjures God against me."

"I shall find him still this day," answered the old woman, "and please God, you shall meet him tomorrow."

With this, the old woman took her leave, went on the same day to the man who had made her his confidant, and told him of the meeting arranged for the next day.

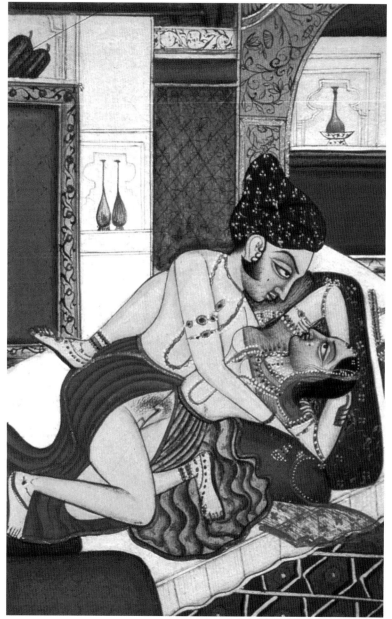

So the next day the mistress of the house went to the old woman, for they had agreed that the rendezvous should take place there. When she arrived at the house, she waited for some time, but the lover did not come. No doubt he had been prevented from making his appearance by some matter of importance.

The old woman, reflecting upon this mischance, thought to herself, "There is no might nor power but in God, the Great." But she could not imagine what might have kept him away. Looking at the woman, she saw that she was agitated, and it was apparent that she wanted coition hotly. She got more and more restless, and presently asked, "Why does he not come?" The old woman made answer, "O my daughter, some serious affair must have interfered, probably necessitating a journey. But I shall help you under these circumstances." She then put on her melahfa, and went to look for the young man. But it was to no purpose, as she could not find out anything about him.

Still continuing her search, the old woman was thinking, "This woman is at this moment eagerly coveting a man. Why not try today another young man, who might calm her ardor? Tomorrow I shall find the right one." As she was thus walking and thinking, she a met a young man of very pleasing exterior. She saw, at once, that he was a fit lover, and likely to help her out of her perplexity; and she spoke to him: O my son, if I were to set you in connection with a lady, beautiful, graceful and perfect, would you make love to her?" "If your words are truth, I would give you this golden dinar!" said he. The old woman, quite enchanted, took the money, and conducted him to her house.

Now, it so happened that this young man was the husband of the lady, which the old woman did not know till she had brought him. And the way she found it out was this: She went first into the house and said to the lady, "I have not been able to find the slightest trace of your lover; but, failing

The beseeching woman

*One of my Syrian mistresses, **Wardah**, was very fair-complexioned. Unlike Muneerah, this one would freeze the moment I penetrated her, and would clasp me with her arms and legs like a baby monkey and not let go. She lay still while I did the work. This continued until she felt her climax; then she would relax her grip, open her thighs wide, and revel in the vaginal contractions that spread through her body.*

At this point, she would begin to toss her head from side to side, groan as if she were suffering terribly, and repeat the word "please" over and over again. After our love-making, I anxiously asked her if she had been in any discomfort; she explained that the pleasure she experienced was so overwhelming that she thought she would die of a heart attack. That was why she begged me to stop. However, she mischievously assured me that she didn't really want me to, of course. The Fountains of Pleasure him, I have brought you somebody to quench your fire for today. We will save the other for tomorrow. God has inspired me to do so."

The lady then went to the window to take a look at him whom the old woman wanted to bring to her, and, getting sight of him, she recognized her husband, just on the point of entering the house. She did not hesitate, but hastily donning her melahfa, she went straight to meet him, and striking him in the face, she exclaimed, "O! enemy of God and of yourself, what are you doing here? You sure came with the intention to commit adultery. I have been suspecting you for a long time, and waited here every day, while I was sending out the old woman to inveigle you to come in. This day I have found you out, and denial is of no use. And you always told me that you were not a rake! I shall demand a divorce this very day, now I know your conduct!"

The husband, believing that his wife spoke the truth, remained silent and abashed.

Learn from this the deceitfulness of woman, and what she is capable of.

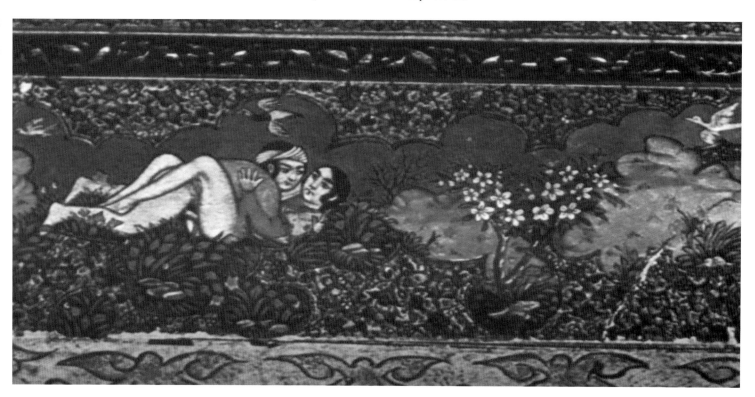

Story of the Lover against his Will

A story is told of a certain woman who was desperately in love with one of her neighbors, whose virtue and piety were well-known. She declared to him her passion; but, finding all her advances constantly repulsed, in spite of all her wiles, she resolved to have her satisfaction nevertheless, and this is the way she went to work her purpose:

On evening she apprised her negress that she intended to set a snare for that man, and the negress, by her order, left the street door open; then, in the middle of the night, she called the negress and gave her the following instructions: "Go and knock with this stone at our street door as hard as you can, without taking any notice of the cries which I shall utter, or the noise I make; as soon as you the the neighbor opening his door, come back and knock the same way at the inner door. Take care that he does not see you, and come in at once if you observe somebody coming." The negress executed this order punctually.

Now, the neighbor was by nature a compassionate man, always disposed to assist people in distress, and his help was never asked in vain. On hearing the noise of the blows struck at the door and the cries of his neighbor, he asked his wife what this might mean, and she replied, "It is our neighbor so and so, who is attacked in her house by thieves." He went in great haste to her aid; but scarcely had he entered the house when the negress closed the door upon him. The woman sized him, and uttered loud screams. He protested, but the mistress of the house put, without any more ado, this condition before him. "If you do not consent to do with me so and so, I shall tell that you have come in here to violate me, and hence all this noise." "The will of God be done!" said the man, "nobody can go against him, nor escape from His might." He then tried sundry subterfuges in order to escape, but in vain, for the mistress of the house recommenced to scream and make a row, which brought a good many people to the spot. He saw that his reputation would compromise if he continued his resistance, and surrendered, saying "Save me, and I am ready to satisfy you!" "Go into this chamber and close the door behind you," said the lady of the house, "if you want to leave this house with honor, and do not attempt escape unless you wish those people to know that you are the author of all this commotion." When he saw how determined she was to have her way, he did as she had told him. She, on her part, went out to the neighbors that had come to help her, and giving them some kind of explanation dismissed them. They went away condoling with her.

Left alone, she shut the doors and returned to her unwilling lover. She kept him in sequestration for a whole week, and only set him free after she had completely drained him.

Learn from this the deceitfulness of women, and what they are capable of.

A Larceny of Love

The following story is told of two women who inhabited the same house. The husband of one of them had a member long, thick and hard; while the husband of the other had, on the contrary, that organ little, insignificant and soft. The first one rose always pleasant and smiling; the other one got up in the morning in tears and veation.

One day the two women were together, and spoke of their husbands.

The first one said, "I live in the greatest happiness. My bed is a couch of bliss. When my husband and I are together in it, it is the witness of our supreme pleasure; of our kisses and embraces, of our joys and amorous signs. When my husband's member is in my vulva it stops it up completely; it stretches itself out until it touches the bottom of my vagina, and it does not take its leave until it has visited every corner – threshold, vestibule, ceiling and center. When the crisis arrives it takes its position in the very center of the vagina, which it floods with tears. It is in this way we quench our fire and appease our passion."

The second answered, :"I live in the greatest grief; our bed is a bed of misery, and our coition is a union of fatigue and trouble, of hate and malediction. When my husband's member enters my vulva there is a space left open, and it is so short it cannot touch the bottom. When it is in erection it is twisted all ways, and cannot procure any pleasure. Feeble and meager, it can scarcely ejaculate a drop, and its service cannot afford pleasure to any woman."

Such was the almost daily conversation, which the two women had together.

It happened, however, that the woman who had so much cause for complaint thought in her heart how delightful it would be to commit adultery with the other one's husband. She thought to herself, "It must be brought about, if it be only for once." Then she watched her opportunity until her husband had to be absent for a night from the house.

In the evening she made preparation to get her project carried out, and perfumed herself with sweet scents and essences. When the night was advanced to about a third of its duration, she noiselessly entered the chamber in which the other woman and her husband were sleeping, and groped her way to their couch. Finding that there was a free space between them, she slipped in. There was a scant room, but each of the spouses thought it was the pressure of the other, and gave way a little; and so she contrived to glide between them. She then quietly waited until the other woman was in a profound sleep, and then, approaching the husband, she brought her flesh in contact with his. He awoke, and smelling the perfumed odors, which she exhaled, he was in erection at once. He drew her towards him, but she said, in a low voice, "Let me go to sleep!" He answered, "Be quiet, and let me do! The children will not hear anything!" She then pressed close up to him, so as to get him farther away from his wife, and said "Do as you like, but do not awaken the children, who are close by." She took these precautions for fear that his wife should wake up.

The man, however, roused by the odor of the perfumes, drew her ardently towards himself. She was plump and mellow, and her vulva projecting. He mounted upon her and said, "Take it" (the member) "in your hand, as usual!" She took it, and was astonished at its size and magnificence, then introduced it into her vulva.

The man, however, observed that his member had been taken in entirely, which he had never been able to do with his wife. The woman, on her part, found that she had never received such a benefit from her husband.

The man was quite surprised. He worked his will upon her a second and third time, but his astonishment only increased. At least he got off her, and stretched himself along her side.

As soon as the woman found that he was asleep, she slipped out, left the chamber, and returned to her own.

In the morning, the husband, on rising, said to his wife, "Your embraces have never seemed so sweet to me as last night, and I never breathed such sweet perfumes as those you exhaled." "What embraces and what perfumes are you speaking of?" asked the wife. "I have not a particle of perfume in the house." She called him a storyteller, and assured him that he must have been dreaming. He then began to consider whether he might not have deceived himself, and agreed with his wife that he must actually have dreamed it all.

Appreciate, after this, the deceitfulness of women, and what they are capable of.

The astonished woman

*Another Syrian girl, **Zulafah**, sweet and naïve, was a voluptuous lover, who moved languorously during intercourse, her legs stretched straight up at right angles to her body. She caressed my body the whole time, and barely detached her mouth, with its fresh roving tongue, from mine.*

I knew she was about to reach orgasm when her rhythm and thrusts accelerated and she lowered her legs and grasped me tightly with them. She would then thrust her pelvis at me at a frenetic pace, and emit a long, deep groan as she surrendered herself to the ecstatic vaginal spasms. The groan turned into a repetition of the word "no", which, she told me subsequently, was an expression of astonishment that such pleasure existed for a woman. She found it hard to believe that she could feel such ecstasy, and was not sure whether this was happening or whether she was only dreaming.

The Fountains of Pleasure

Story of the Woman with Two Husbands

It is related that a man, after having lived for some time in a country to which he had gone, became desirous of getting married. He addressed himself to an old woman who had experience in such matter, asking her whether she could find him a wife, and she replied, "I can find you a girl gifted with great beauty, and perfect in shape and comeliness. She will

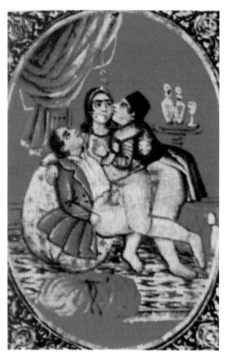

surely suit you, for besides having these qualities, she is virtuous and pure. Only mark, her business occupies her all the day, but during the night she will be yours completely. It is for this reason she keeps herself reserved, as she apprehends that a husband might not agree to this."

The man replied, "This girl need not be afraid. I, too, am not at liberty during the day, and I only want her for the night."

He then asked her in marriage. The old woman brought her to him and he liked her. From that time they lived together, observing the conditions under which they had come together.

This man had an intimate friend whom he introduced to the old woman who had arranged his marriage according to the conditions mentioned, and which friend had requested the man to ask her to do him the same service. They went to the old woman and solicited her assistance in the matter. "This is a very easy matter," she said. "I know a girl of great beauty, who will dissipate your heaviest troubles. Only the business she is carrying on keeps her at work all night, but she will be with your friend all day long." "This shall be no hindrance." Replied the friend. She then brought the young girl to him. He was well-pleased with her, and married her on the conditions agreed upon.

But before long the two friends found out that the two wives, which the old harridan had procured for them were only one woman.

Appreciate, after this, the deceitfulness of women, and what they are capable of.

Story of Bahia

It is related that a married woman of the name of Bahia (splendid beauty) had a lover whose relations to her were soon a mystery to no one, for which reason she had to leave him. Her absence affected him to such a degree that he fell ill, because he could not see her.

One day he went to see one of his friends, and said to him, "Oh, my brother! An ungovernable desire has seized me, and I can wait no more. Could you accompany me on a visit I am going to pay to Bahia, the well-beloved of my hear?" The friend declared himself willing.

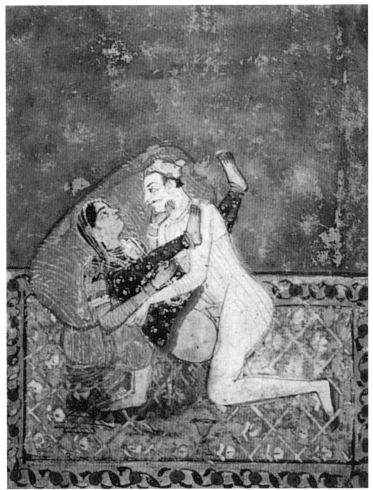

The next day they mounted their horses; and after a journey of two days, they arrived near the place where Bahia dwelt. There they stopped. The lover said to his friend, "Go and see the people that live about here, and ask for their hospitality, but take good care not to divulge our intentions, and try in particular to find the servant girl of Bahia, to whom you can say that I am here, and whom you will charge with the message to her mistress that I would like to see her." He then described the servant-maid to him.

The friend went, met the servant, and told her all that was necessary. She went at once to Bahia, and repeated to her what she had been told.

Bahia sent to the friend the message, "Inform him who sent you that the meeting will take place tonight, near such and such a tree, at such and such an hour."

Returning to the lover, the friend communicated to him the decision of Bahia about the rendezvous.

At the hour that had been fixed, the two friends were near to the tree. They had not to wait long for Bahia. As soon as her lover saw her coming, he rushed to meet her, kissed her, pressed her to his heart, and they began to embrace and caress each other.

The lover said to her, "O Bahia, is there no way to enable us to pass the night together without rousing the suspicions of your husband?" She answered, "Oh, before God! If it will give you pleasure, the means to contrive this are not wanting." "Hasten," said her lover, "to let me know how it may be done." She then asked him "Your friend here, is he devoted to you, and intelligent!" He answered, "Yes," She then rose, too off her garments, and handed them to the friend, who gave her his, in which she then dressed herself; then she made the friend put on her clothes. The lover said, surprised, "What are you going to do?" "Be silent," she answered, and addressing herself to the friend, she gave him the following explanations: "Go to my house and lie down in my bed. After a third part of the night is passed, my husband will come to you and ask you for the pot into which they milk the camels. You will then take up the vase, but you must keep it in your hands until he takes it from you. This is our usual way. Then he will go and return with the pot filled with milk, and say to you, "Here is the pot!" But you must not take it from him until he has repeated these words. Then take it out of his hands, or let him put it on the ground himself. After that, you will not see anything more of

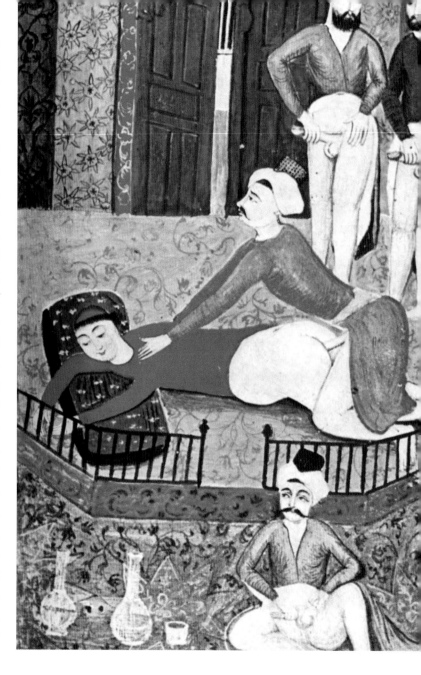

him till the morning. After the pot has been put on the ground, and my husband is gone, drink the third part of the milk, and replace the pot on the ground."

The friend went, observed all these recommendations, and when the husband returned with the pot full of milk he did not take it out of his hands until he had said twice, "Here is the pot"! Unfortunately he withdrew his hands when the husband was going to set it down, the latter thinking the pot was being held, let it go, and the vase fell upon the ground and was broken. The husband, in the belief that he was speaking to his wife, exclaimed, "What have you been thinking of?" and beat him with a switch till it broke; then took another, and continued to batter him stroke on stroke enough to break his back. The mother and sister of Bahia came running to the spot to tear her from his hands. He had fainted. Luckily they succeeded in getting the husband away.

The mother of Bahia soon came back, and talked to him so long that he was fairly sick of her talk; but he could do nothing but be silent and weep. At last she finished, saying "Have confidence in God, and obey your husband. As for your lover, he cannot come now to see and console you, but I will send your sister to keep you company." And so she went away.

She did send, indeed, the sister of Bahia, who began to console her and curse him who had beaten her. He felt his heart warming towards her, for he had seen that she was of resplendent beauty, endowed with all perfections, and like the full moon in the night. He placed his hand over her mouth, so as to prevent her from speaking, and said to her, "O, lady! I am not what you think. Your sister Bahia is at present with her lover, and I have run into danger to do her a service. Will you not take me under your protection? If you denounce me, your sister will be covered with shame; as for me, I have done my part, but the evil may fall back upon you!"

The young girl then began to tremble like a leaf, in thinking of the consequences of her sister's doings, and then, beginning to laugh, surrendered herself to the friend who had proved himself so true. They passed the remainder of the night in bliss, kisses, embraces, and mutual enjoyment. He found her the best of the best. In her arms he forgot the beating he had received, and they did not cease to play, toy, and make love till daybreak.

He then returned to his companion. Bahia asked him how he had fared, and he said to her, "Ask your sister. By my faith! She knows it all! Only know, that we have passed in the night in mutual pleasure, kissing and enjoying ourselves until now."

Then they changed clothes again, each one taking his own, and the friend told Bahia all the particulars of what had happened to him.

Appreciate, after this, the deceitfulness of women, and what they are capable of.

The Story of the Man Who Was an Expert in Stratagems, and Was Duped by a Woman

A story is told of a man who had studied all the ruses and all the stratagems invented by women for the deception of men, and boasted that no woman could dupe him.

A woman of great beauty, and full of charms, got to hear of his conceit. She, therefore, prepared for him in the medjeles a collation, in which several kinds of wine figured, and nothing was wanting in the way of rare and choice viands. Then she sent for him, and invited him to come and see her. As she was famed for her great beauty and the rare perfection of her person, she had roused his desires, and he made haste to avail himself of her invitation.

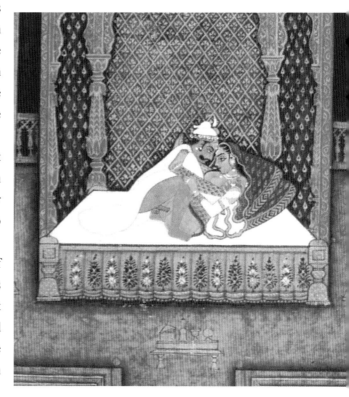

She was dressed in her finest garments, and exhaled the choicest perfumes, and assuredly whoever had thus seen her would have been troubled in his mind. And thus, when he was admitted into her presence, he was fascinated by her charms, and plunged into admiration of her marvelous beauty.

This woman, however, appeared to be preoccupied on account of her husband, and allowed it to be seen that she was afraid of his coming back from one minute to another. It must be mentioned that this husband was very proud, very jealous and very violent, and would not have hesitated to shed the blood of anyone whom he would have found prowling about his house. What would he have done, and, with much more reason, to the man whom he might have found inside!

While the lady and he who flattered himself that he should possess her were amusing themselves in the medjeles, a knock at the house-door filled the lover with fear and trouble, particularly when the lady cried, "This is my husband, who is returning." All in a tremble, she hid him in a closet, which was in the room, shut the door upon him, and left the key in the medjeles; then she opened the house-door.

Her husband, for it was he, saw, on entering, the wine and all the preparations that had been made. Surprised, he asked what this meant. "It means what you see," she answered. "But for whom is all this?" he asked.

It is for my lover whom I have here."

And where is he?"

"in this closet," she said, pointing with her finger to the place where the sufferer was confined.

At these words the husband started. He rose and went to the closet, but found it locked. "Where is the key?" he said. She answered, "Here!" throwing it to him. But as he was putting it into the lock she burst out laughing uproariously. He turned towards her, and said, "What are you laughing at?" "I laugh," she answered, "at the weakness of your judgment, and your want of reason and reflection. Oh, you man without sense, do you think that if I had in reality a lover, and had admitted him into this room, I should have told you that he was here and where he was hidden? That is certainly not likely. I had no other thought than to offer you a collation on your return, and wanted only to have a joke with you in doing as I did. If I had had a lover, I should certainly not have mad you my confidant."

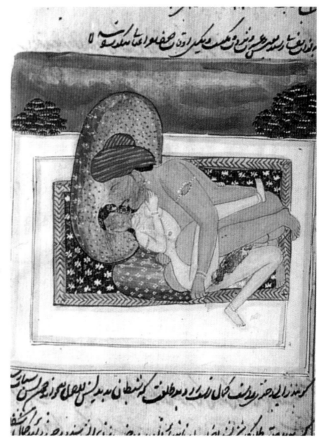

The husband left the key in the lock of the closet without having turned it, returned to the table, and said, "True! I rose; but I have not the slightest doubt about the sincerity of your words." Then they ate and drank together, and made love.

The man in the closet had to stop there until the husband went out. Then the lady went to set him free, and found him quite undone and in a bad state. When he came out, after having escaped an imminent peril, she said to him, "Well, you wiseacre, who know so well the stratagems of women, of all those you know, is there one to equal this?" He made answer, "I am now convinced that your stratagems are countless."

Appreciate after this the deceits of woman, and what they are capable of.

Story of the Lover Who was Surprised by the Unexpected Arrival of the Husband

It is related that a woman who was married to a violent and brutal man, having her lover with her on the unexpected arrival of her husband, who was returning from a journey, had only just time to hide him under the bed. She was compelled to let him remain in this dangerous and unpleasant position, knowing of no experiment which might enable him to leave the house. In her restlessness she went to and fro, and having gone to the street door, one of her neighbors, a woman, saw that she was in trouble, and asked her the reason of it. She told her what had happened. The other then said, "Return into the house. I will charge myself with the safety of your lover, and I promise you that he shall come out unharmed." Then the woman re-entered her house.

Her neighbor was not long in joining her, and together they prepared the meal, and then they all sat down to eat and drink. The woman sat facing her husband, and the neighbor opposite the bed. The latter began to tell stories and anecdotes about the tricks of women; and the lover under the bed heard all that was going on.

Pursuing her tales, the neighbor told the following one: "A married woman had a lover, whom she loved tenderly, and by whom she was equally loved. One day the lover came to see her in the absence of her husband. But the latter happened to return home unexpectedly just as they were together. The woman, knowing of no better place, hid her lover under the bed, then sat down by her husband, who was taking some refreshment, and joked and played with him. Among other playful games, she covered her husband's eyes with a napkin, and her lover took this opportunity to come out from under the bed and escape unobserved."

The wife understood at once how to profit by this tale; taking a napkin and covering the eyes of her husband with it, she said, "Then it was by means of this ruse that the lover was helped out of hi dilemma." And the lover, taking the opportunity, succeeded in making good his escape unobserved by the husband. Unconscious of what had happened this latter laughed at the story, and his merriment was still increased by the last words of his wife and by her action.

Appreciate after this the deceitfulness of women, and what they are capable of.

The Perfumed Garden of the Sheikh Nefzaoui

Chapter 12

Concerning Sundry Observations Useful to Know for Men and Women

Know, O Vizir (to whom God be good!), that the information contained in this chapter is of the greatest utility, and it is only in this book that such can be found. Assuredly to know things is better than to be ignorant of them. Knowledge may be bad, but ignorance is still more so.

The knowledge in question concerns matters unknown to you, and relating to women.

There was once a woman, name Moarbeda, who was considered to be the most knowing and wisest person of her time. She was a philosopher. One day various queries were put to her, and among them the following, which I shall give here, with her answers.

"In what part of a woman's body does her mind reside?"

"Between her thighs."

"And where her enjoyment?"

"In the same place."

"And where the love of men and the hatred of them?"

"In the vulva," she said, adding, "To the man whom we love we give our vulva, and we refuse it to him we hate. We share our property with the man we love, and are content with whatever little he may be able to bring to us; if he has no fortune, we take him as he is. But, on the other hand, we keep at a distance him whom we hate, were he to offer us wealth and riches."

"Where, in a woman, are located knowledge, love and taste?"

"In the eye, the heart, and the vulva."

When asked for explanation on this subject, she replied: "Knowledge dwells in the eye, for it is the woman's eye that appreciates the beauty of form and of appearance. By the medium of this organ, love penetrates into the heart and dwells in it, and enslaves it. A woman in love pursues the object of her love, and lays snares for it. If she succeeds, there will be an encounter between the beloved one and her vulva. The vulva tastes him and then knows his sweet or bitter flavor. It is, in fact, the vulva which knows how to distinguish, by tasting, the good from the bad."

"Which virile members are preferred by women? What women are most eager for coitus, and which are those who detest it? Which are the men preferred by women, and which are those whom they abominate?"

She answered, "Not all women have the same conformation of vulva, and they also different in heir manner of making love, and in their love for and their aversion to things. The same disparities exist in men, both with regard to their organizes and their tastes. A woman of plump form and with a shallow uterus will look out for a member which is both short and thick, which will completely fill her vagina, without touching the bottom of it; a long and large member would not suit her. A woman with a deep lying uterus, and consequently a long vagina, only yearns for a member which is long and thick and of ample proportions, and thus fills her vagina in its whole extension; she will despise the man with a small and slender member for he could never satisfy her in coition.

"The following distinctions exists in the temperaments of women: the bilious, the melancholy, the sanguine, the phlegmatic, and the mixed. Those with a bilious or melancholy temperament are not much given to coitus, and like it only with men of the same disposition. Those who are sanguine or phlegmatic love coition to excess, and if they encounter a member, they would never let it leave their vulva if they could help it. With these also it is only men of

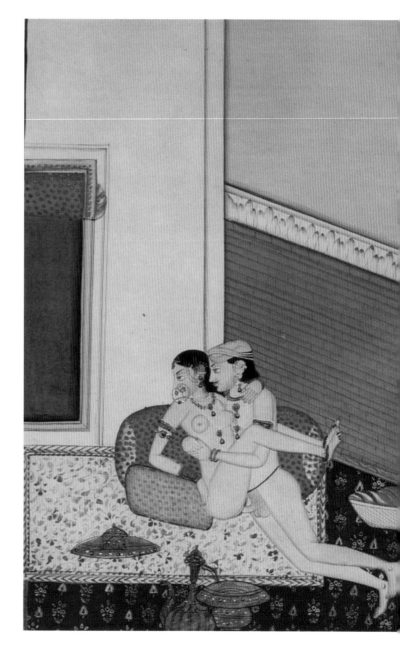

their own temperament who can satisfy them, and if such a woman were married to a bilious or melancholy man, they would lead a sorry life together. As regards mixed temperaments, they exhibit neither a marked predilection for, nor aversion against coitus.

"It has been observed that under all circumstances little women love coitus more and evince a stronger affection for the virile member than women of a large size. Only long and vigorous members suit them; in them they find the delight of their existence and of their couch.

"There are also women who love the coitus only on the edge of their vulva, and when a man lying upon them wants to get his member into the vagina, they take it out with the hand and place its gland between the lips of the vulva."

I have every reason to believe that this is only the case with young girls or with women not used to women. I pray God to preserve us from such, or from women for whom it is a matter of impossibility to give themselves up to men.

"There are women who will do their husband's behests, and will satisfy them and give them voluptuous pleasure by coition, only if compelled by blows and ill-treatment. Some people ascribe this conduct to the aversion they feel either against coition or against the husband; but this is not so; it is simply a question of temperament and character.

"There are also women who do not care for coition because all their ideas turn upon the grandeurs, personal honors, ambitious hopes, or business cares of the world.

The talkative woman

One of my wives was a petite but beautifully proportioned Yemenite girl with perfect skin called **Haneefah**. *She was a sweet, shy, quiet girl who only spoke when I addressed her – and then responded minimally and respectfully.*

While she had a surprisingly large vulva for her size, her vagina was narrow and tight. She remained completely silent during our foreplay, but knew exactly what to do to please me, since she had been an apt pupil.

All her bashfulness and respectful silence disappeared in a flash the moment I penetrated her. A stream of gentle affectionate words would gush from her mouth unceasingly – words of adoration and encouragement – and she would meet my thrusts enthusiastically.

When her climax began, she would like still, close her thighs and squeeze them together rhythmically and give me loving but demanding instructions: "Oh, Master, please don't stop… faster, please… I love you…" and things to that effect. This would go on until the last spasm had faded away. Her orgasms usually lasted twenty seconds.

At this point, she reopened her thighs to allow me to plunge deeply inside her, and would always thank me in the most ardent terms. The Fountains of Pleasure

With others this indifference springs, as it may be, from purity of the heart, or from jealousy, or from a pronounced tendency of their souls towards another world, or lastly from past violent sorrow. Furthermore, the pleasures which they feel in coition depend not alone upon the size of the member, but also upon the particular conformation of their own natural parts. Among those the vulva called from its form el morteba, the square one, and el mortafa, the projecting, is remarkable. This vulva has the peculiarity of projecting all round when the woman is standing up and closes her thighs. It burns for the coitus, its slit is narrow, and it is also called el keulihimi, the pressed one. The woman who has such a one likes only large members, and they must not let her wait long for the crisis. But this is a general characteristic of women.

"As to the desire of men for coition, I must say that they also are addicted to it more or less according to their different temperaments, five in number, like the women's, with the difference that the hankering of the woman after the member is stronger than that of the man after the vulva.

"What are the faults of women?"

Moarbeda replied to this question, "The worst of women is she who immediately cries out aloud as soon as her husband wants to touch the smallest amount of her property for his necessities. In the same line stands she who divulges matters which her husband wants to be kept secret."

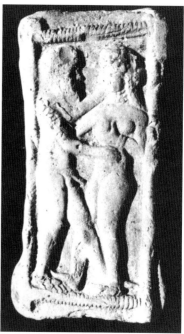

"Are there any more?" she is asked. She adds, "The woman of a jealous disposition and the woman who raises her voice so as to drown that of her husband; she who disseminates scandal; the woman that scowls; the one who is always burning to let men see her beauty, and cannot stay at home; and with respect to this last let me add that a woman who laughs much, and is constantly seen at the street door, may be taken to be an arrant prostitute.

"Bad also are those women who mind people's affairs; those who are always complaining; those who steal things belonging to their husbands; those of a disagreeable and imperious temper; those who are not grateful for kindnesses received; those that will not share the conjugal couch, or who incommode their husbands by the uncomfortable positions they take in it; those who are inclined to deceit, treachery, calumny and ruse.

"Then there are still women who are unlucky in whatever they undertake; those who are always inclined to blame and censure; those who invite their husbands to fulfill their conjugal duty only when it is convenient for them; those that make noises in bed; and lastly those who are shameless, without intelligence, tattlers and curious.

"Here you have the worst specimens among women."

The Perfumed Garden of the Sheikh Nefzaoui

Concerning the Causes of Enjoyment in the Act of Generation

Know, O Vizir (to whom God be good!) that the causes which tend to develop the passion for coition are six in number: the fire of an ardent love, the superabundance of sperm, the proximity of the loved person whose possession is eagerly desired, the beauty of the face, exciting viands, and contact.

Know also, that the causes of the pleasure in cohabitation, and the conditions of enjoyment are numerous, but that the principal and best ones are: the heat of the vulva; the narrowness, dryness, and sweet exhalation of the same. If any one of these conditions is absent, there is at the same time something wanting in the voluptuous enjoyment. But if the vagina unites the required qualification, the enjoyment is complete. In fact, a moist vulva relaxes the nerves, a cold one robs the member of all its vigor, and bad exhalations from the vagina detract greatly from the pleasure, as is also the case if the latter is very wide.

The acme of enjoyment, which is produced by the abundance and impetuous ejaculation of the sperm, depends upon one circumstance, and this is, that the vulva is furnished with a suction-pump (orifice of the uterus), which will clasp the virile member, and suck up the sperm with an irresistible force. The member once seized by the orifice, the lover is powerless to retain the sperm, for the orifice will not relax its hold until it has extracted every drop of the sperm, and certainly if the crisis arrives before this gripping of the glad takes place, the pleasure of the ejaculation will not be complete.

Know that there are eight things which give strength to and favor the ejaculation. These are: bodily health, the absence of all care and worry, and unembarrassed mind, natural gaiety of spirit, good nourishment, wealth, the variety of women, and the variety of the complexions.

If you wish to acquire strength for coitus, take fruit of the mastic tree (derou), pound them and macerate them with oil and honey; then drink of the liquid first thing in the morning: you will thus become vigorous for the coitus, and there will be abundance of sperm produced.

The same result will be obtained by rubbing the virile member and the vulva with gall from the jackal. This rubbing stimulates those parts and increases their vigor.

A savant of the name of Djelinouss has said: "He who feels that he is weak for coition should drink before going to bed a glassful of very thick honey and eat twenty almonds and one hundred grains of the pine tree. He must follow this regime for three days. He may also pound onion seed, sift it and mix it afterwards with honey, stirring the mixture well, and take of this mixture while still fasting."

A man who would wish to acquire vigor for coition may likewise melt down fat from the hump of a camel, and rub his member with it just before the act; it will then perform wonders, and the woman will praise it for its work.

If you would make the enjoyment still more voluptuous, masticate a little cubeb-pepper or cardamom grains of the large species; put a certain quantity of it upon the head of your member, and then go to work. This will procure for you, as well as for the woman, a matchless enjoyment. The ointment from the balm of Judea or of Mecca produces a similar effect.

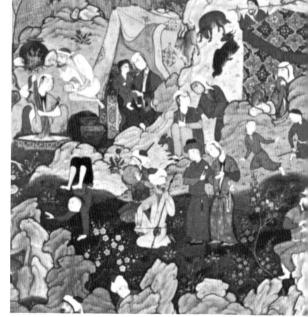

If you would make yourself very strong for the coitus, pound very carefully pyrether together with ginger, mix them while pounding with ointment of lilac, then rub with this compound your abdomen, the testicles, and the verge. This will make you ardent for coitus.

You will likewise predispose yourself for cohabitation, sensibly increase the volume of your sperm, gain increased vigor for the action, and procure for yourself extraordinary erections, by eating of chrysocolla the size of a mustard grain. The excitement resulting from the use of this nostrum is unparalleled, and all your qualifications for coitus will be increased.

If you wish the woman to be inspired with a great desire to cohabit with you, take a little of cubebs, pyrether, ginger and cinnamon, which you will have to masticate just before joining her; then moisten your member with your saliva and do her business for her. From that moment she will have such an affection for you that she can scarcely be a moment without you.

The virile member, rubbed with ass's milk, will become uncommonly strong and vigorous.

Green peas, boiled carefully with onion, and powdered with cinnamon, ginger and cardamoms, well pounded, create for the consumer considerable amorous passion and strength in coitus.

The Perfumed Garden of the Sheikh Nefzaoui

Description of the Uterus of Sterile Women, and Treatment of the Same

Know, O Vizir (God be good to you!) that wise physicians have plunged into this sea of difficulties to very little purpose. Each one has looked at the matter from his own point of view, and in the end the question has been left in the dark.

Among the causes which determine the sterility of women may be taken the obstruction of the uterus by clots of blood, the accumulation of water, the want of or defective sperm of the man, organic malformation of the parts of the latter, internal defects in the uterus, stagnation of the courses and the corruption of the menstrual fluid, and the habitual presence of wind in the uterus. Other savants attribute the sterility of women to the action of spirits and spells. Sterility is common in women who are very corpulent, so that their uterus gets compressed and cannot conceive, not being able to take up the sperm, especially if the husband's member is short and his testicles afre very fat; in such a case the act of copulation can only be imperfectly completed.

One of the remedies against sterility consists of the marrow from the hump of a camel, which the woman spreads on a piece of linen, and rubs her sexual parts with, after having been purified subsequently to her courses. To complete the cure, she takes some fruits of the plant called "jackal's grapes," squeezes the juice out of them into a vase, and then adds a little vinegar; of this medicine she drinks, fasting for seven days, during which time her husband will take care to have copulation with her.

The woman may besides pound a small quantity of sesame grain and mix its juice with a bean's weight of sandarach powder; of this mixture she drinks during three days after her periods; she is then fit to receive her husband's embraces.

The first of these beverages is to be taken separately, and in the first instance; if this the second, which will have a salutary effect, if so it pleases the Almighty God!

There is still another remedy. A mixture is made of nitre, gall from a sheep or a cow, a small quantity of the plant named el meusk, and of the grains of that plant. The woman saturates a plug of soft wool with this mixture, and rubs her vulva with it after menstruation; she then receives the caresses of her husband, and, with the will of God the Highest, will become pregnant

The Perfumed Garden of the Sheikh Nefzaoui

Chapter 15

Concerning the Causes of Impotence in Men

Know, O Vizir (God be good to you!) that there are men whose sperm is vitiated by the inborn coldness of their nature, by the diseases of their organs, by the purulent discharges, and by fevers. There are also men with the urinary canal in their verge deviating owing to a downward curve; the result of such conformation that the seminal liquid cannot be ejected in a straight direction, but falls downwards.

Other men have the member too short or too small to reach the neck of the matrix, or their bladder is ulcerated, or they are affected by other infirmities, which prevent them from coition.

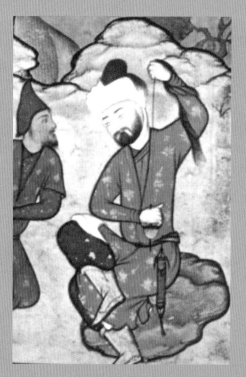

Finally, there are men who arrive quicker at the crisis than women, is consequence of which the two emissions are not simultaneous; there is in such cases no conception.

All these circumstances serve to explain the absence of conception in women; but the principal cause of all is the shortness of the virile member.

As another cause of impotence may be regarded the sudden transmission from hot to cold, and vice versa, and a great number of analogous reasons.

Men whose impotence is due either to the corruption of their sperm owing to their cold nature, or to maladies of the organs, or to discharges or fevers and similar ills, or to their excessive promptness in ejaculation, can be cured. They should eat stimulant pastry containing honey, ginger, pyrether, syrup of vinegar, hellebore, garlic, cinnamon, nutmeg, cardamoms, sparrows' tongues, Chinese cinnamon, long pepper, and other spices. They will be cured by using them.

As to the other afflictions which we have indicated – the curvature of the urethra, the small dimension of the virile member, ulcers on the bladder, and the other infirmities which are adverse to coition – God only can cure them.

The Perfumed Garden of the Sheikh Nefzaoui

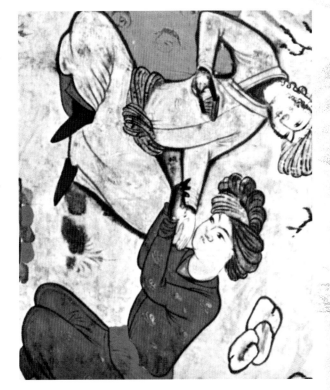

I drank, but the draught of his glance, not wine;
And his swaying gait swayed to sleep these eyne [eyes]:
'Twas not grape-juice gript me but grasp of Past
'Twas not bowl o'erbowled me but gifts divine:
His coiling curl-lets [little curls] my soul ennetted [captured]
And his cruel will all my wits outwitted. *The Arabian Nights*

Chapter 16

Undoing of Aiguillettes (Impotence for a Time)

Know, O Vizir (God be good to you!) that impotence arises from three causes:

Firstly, from the typing of aiguillettes.

Secondly, from a feeble and relaxed constitution.

And thirdly, from too premature ejaculation.

To cure the typing of aiguillettes you must take galanga, cinnamon from Mecca, cloves, Indian cachou, nutmeg, Indian cubebs, sparrowwort, cinnamon, Persian pepper, Indian thistle, cardamoms, pyrether, laurel seed, and gilly flowers. All these ingredients must be pounded together carefully, and one drinks of it as much as one can, morning and night, in broth, particularly in pigeon broth; fowl broth may, however, be substituted just as well. Water is to be drunk before and after taking it. The compound may likewise be taken with honey, which is the best method, and gives the best results.

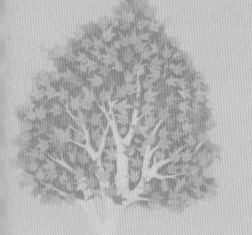

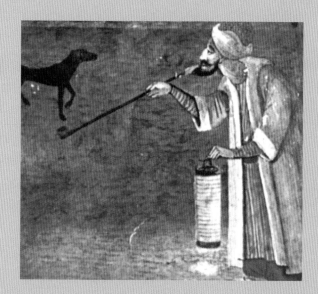

The man whose ejaculation is too precipitate must take nutmeg and incense (oliban) mixed together with honey.

If the impotence arises from weakness, the following ingredients are to be taken in honey: viz., pyrether, nettleseed, a little spurge (or cevadille), ginger, cinnamon of Mecca, and cardamom. This preparation will cause the weakness to disappear and effect the cure, with the permission of God the Highest!

I can warrant the efficacy of all these preparations, the virtue of which has been tested.

The impossibility of performing the coitus, owing to the absence of stiffness in the member, is also due to other causes. It will happen, for instance, that a man with his verge in erection will find it getting flaccid just when he is on the point of introducing it between the thighs of the woman. He thinks this is impotence, while it is simply the result, maybe of an exaggerated respect for the woman, may be of a misplaced bashfulness, may be because one has observed something disagreeable, or on account of an unpleasant odor; finally, owing to a feeling of jealousy, inspired by the reflection that the woman is no longer a virgin, and has served the pleasures of other men.

The Perfumed Garden of the Sheikh Nefzaoui

Mine eyes were dragomans [interpreters] for my tongue betied [paralysed]
And told full clear the love I fain would [was eager to] hide:
When last we met and tears in torrents railed [flowed]
For tongue struck dumb my glances testified:
She signed with eye-glance while her lips were mute
I signed with fingers and she keened [understood] th' implied:
Our eyebrows did all duty 'twixt us twain [between the two of us]:
And we being speechless Love spake loud and plain. *The Arabian Nights*

Prescription for Increasing the Dimension of Small Members and for Making Them Splendid

Know, O Vizir (God be good to you!) that this chapter, which treats of the size of the virile member, is of the first importance both for men and women. For the men because from a good sized and vigorous member there springs the affection and love of women; for the women; because it is by such members that their amorous passions are appeased, and the greatest pleasure is procured for them. This is evident from the fact that many men, solely by reason of their insignificant members, are, as far as coition is concerned, objects of aversion to women, who likewise entertain the same sentiment with regard to those whose members are soft, nerveless, and relaxed. Their whole happiness consists in the use of robust and strong members.

A man, therefore, with a small member, who wants to make it grand or fortify it for the coitus, must rub it before copulation with tepid water, until it gets red and extended by the blood flowing into it, in consequence of the heat; he must then anoint it with a mixture of honey and ginger, rubbing it in sedulously. The let him join the woman; he will procure for her such pleasure that she objects to him getting off her again.

Another remedy consists of a compound made of a moderate quantity of pepper, lavender, galanga, and musk, reduced to powder, sifted, and mixed up with honey and preserved ginger. The member, after having been first washed in warm water, is then vigorously rubbed with the mixture; it will then grow large and brawny, and afford to the woman a marvelous feeling of voluptuousness.

A third remedy is the following: wash the member in water until it becomes red, and enters into erection. Then take a piece of soft leather, upon which spread hot pitch, and envelop the member with it. It will not be long before the member raises its head, trembling with passion. The leather is to be left on until the pitch grows cold, and the member is again in a state of repose. This operation, several times repeated, will have the effect of making the member strong and thick.

A fourth remedy is based upon the use made of leeches, but only of such as live in water (sic). You put as many of them into a bottle as can be got in, and fill it up with oil. Then expose the bottle to the sun, until the heat of the same has effected a complete mixture. With the fluid thus obtained the member is to e rubbed several consecutive days, and it will by being thus treated, become of a good size and of full dimensions.

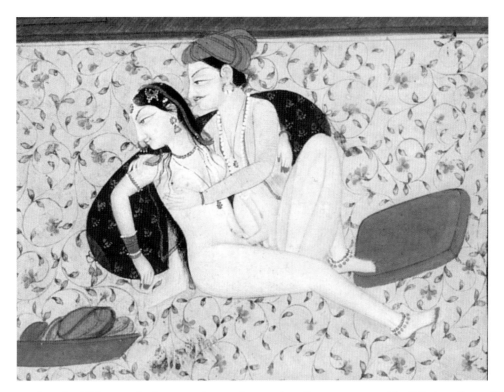

For another procedure I will here note the use of an ass's member. Procure one and boil it, together with onions and a large quantity of corn. With this dish feed fowls, which you eat afterwards. One can also macerate the ass's verge in oil, and use the fluid thus obtained for anointing one's member, and drinking of it.

Another way is to bruise leeches with oil, and rub the verge with this ointment; or, if it is preferred, the leeches may be put into a bottle, and, thus enclosed, buried in a warm dung-hill until they are dissolved into a coherent mass and form a sort of liniment, which is used for repeatedly anointing the member. The member is certain greatly to benefit by this.

One may likewise take rosin and wax, mixed with tubipore, asphodel, and cobbler's glue, with which mixture rub the member, and the result will be that its dimensions will be enlarged.

The efficacy of all these remedies is well-known, and I have tested them.

The Perfumed Garden of the Sheikh Nefzaoui

Chapter 18

Of Things that Take Away the Bad Smell from the Armpits and Sexual Parts of Women and Contract the Latter

Know, O Vizir (God be good to you!) that bad exhalations from the vulva and from the armpits are, as is also a wide vagina, the greatest of evils.

If a woman wants this bad odor to disappear she must pound red myrrh, then sift it, and knead this powder with myrtle-water, and rub her sexual parts with this wash. All disagreeable emanation will disappear from her vulva.

Another remedy is obtained by pounding lavender, and kneading it afterwards with musk-rose water. Saturate a piece of woolen stuff with it, and rub the vulva with the same until it is hot. The bad smell will be removed by this.

If a woman intends to contract her vagina, she has only to dissolve alum in water, and wash her sexual parts with the solution, which may be made still more efficacious by the addition of a little bark of the walnut tree, the latter substance being very astringent.

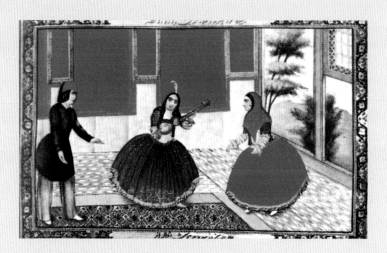

Another remedy to be mentioned is the following, which is well-known for its efficacy. Boil well in water carobs (locusts), freed from their kernels, and bark of the pomegranate tree. The woman takes a sitz bath in the decoction thus obtained, which must be as hot as she can bear it; when the bath gets cold, it must be warmed and used again, and this immersion is to be repeated several times. The same result may be obtained by fumigating the vulva with cow-dung.

To do away with the bad smell of the armpits, one takes antimony and mastic, which are to be pounded together, and put with water into an earthen vase. The mixture is then rubbed against the sides of the vase until it turns red; when it is ready for use, rub it into the armpits, and the bad smell will be removed. It must be used repeatedly, until a radical cure is effected. The same result may be arrived at by pounding together antimony (hadida) and mastic, setting the mixture afterwards on to a stove over a low fire, until it is of the consistency of bread, and rubbing the residue with a stone until the pellicle, which will have formed, is removed. Then rub it into the armpits, and you may be sure that the bad smell will soon be gone.

The Perfumed Garden of the Sheikh Nefzaoui

The agonized woman

I was given Lala, a Berber slave, as a gift by a man of high station who was my employer. She was a big woman with blue eyes and a pale skin. While she was not particularly young – she was thirty when I received her – she looked good and her health was excellent.

As soon as we began to make love, her legs would open wide and she would breathe deeply and convulsively. When I heard the deep grunting sounds issuing from her throat, I knew that she had reached her climax. The pallor of her face became suffused with crimson, and it looked as if she were suffocating. As her vagina pulsed, her arms and legs held and released me in turn. Her frightening sounds would last for the entire duration of her orgasm – some fifteen or twenty seconds – at which point she would pass out completely, her face becoming deathly pale and her hands and feet ice cold. This would last for a few minutes.

I was anxious that this state of unconsciousness had been induced by pain or suffering of some kind, but when I asked her, she was astonished, and replied that on the contrary – it was the unbearable intensity of the pleasure and ecstasy that caused her to pass out.

Once she had recovered from her moments of unconsciousness, she was ready to go again, and it did not take much coaxing on her part to get me excited once again.

The Fountains of Pleasure

Instructions with Regard to Pregnancy and How the Gender of the Child That is to be Born May be Known – that is to say, Knowledge of the Sex of the Fetus

Know, O Vizir (God be good to you!) that the certain indications of pregnancy are the following: the dryness of the vulva immediately after coitus, the inclination to stretch herself, accesses of somnolency, heavy and profound sleep, the frequent contraction of the opening of the vulva to such an extent that not even a meroud could penetrate, the nipples of the breast becoming darker and, lastly, the most certain of all marks is the cessation of menstruation.

If the woman remains always in good health from the time that her pregnancy is certain, if she preserves the good looks of her face and a clear complexion, if hse does not become freckled, then it may be taken as a sign that the child will be a boy.

The red color of the nipples also points to a child of the male sex. The strong development of the breasts, and bleeding from the nose, if it comes from the right nostril, are signs of the same purport.

The signs pointing to the conception of a child of the female sex are numerous. I will name them here: frequent indisposition during pregnancy, pale complexion, spots and freckles, pains in the matrix, frequent nightmares, blackness of the nipples, a heavy feeling on the left side, nasal hemorrhage on the same side.

If there is any doubt about the pregnancy, let the woman drink, on going to bed, honey-water, and if then she has a feeling of heaviness in the abdomen, it is proof that she is with child. If the right side feels heavier than the left one, it will be a boy. If the breasts are swelling with milk, this is similarly a sign that the child she is bearing will be of the male sex.

I have received this information from savants, and all the indications are positive and tested.

The Perfumed Garden of the Sheikh Nefzaoui

Tale of the First Eunuch, Bukhyat.

Know, O my brothers, that when I was a little one, some five years old, I was taken home from my native country by a slave-driver who sold me to a certain Apparitor [royal messenger]. My purchaser had a daughter three years old, with whom I was brought up, and they used to make mock of me, letting me play with her and dance for her and sing to her, till I reached the age of twelve and she that of ten; and even then they did not forbid me seeing her. One day I went in to her and found her sitting in an inner room, and she looked as if she had just come out of the bath which was in the house; for she was scented with essences and reek [perfume] of aromatic woods, and her face shone like the circle of the moon on the fourteenth night. She began to sport with me, and I with her, till, before I knew what I did, I did away her maidenhead. When I saw this, I ran off and took refuge with one of my comrades. Presently her mother came in to her; and seeing her in this case [condition], fainted clean away. However she managed the matter advisedly and hid it from the girl's father out of good will to me; nor did they cease to call to me and coax me, till they took me from where I was. After two months had passed, her mother married her to a young man, a barber who used to shave her papa, and portioned [gave her a dowry] and fitted her out of her own monies; whilst the father knew nothing of what had passed. On the night of the consummation they cut the throat of a pigeon-poult [a young pigeon] and sprinkled the blood on her shift. After a while they seized me unawares and gelded [castrated] me, and, when they brought her to her bridegroom, they made me her Agha [sir], her eunuch, to walk before her wheresoever she went, whether to the bath or to her father's house. I abode [lived] with her a long time enjoying her beauty and loveliness by way of kissing and coupling with her, till she died, and her husband and mother and father died also; when they seized me for the Royal Treasury as being the property of an intestate, and I found my way hither, where I became your comrade. This, then, O my brethren, is the cause of my cullions [testicles] being cut off; and peace be with you!

The Arabian Nights

Forming the Conclusion of this Work and Treating of the Good Effects of the Deglutition of Eggs as Favorable to the Coitus

Know, O Vizir (God be good to you!) that this chapter contains the most useful instructions – how to increase the intensity of the coitus – and that the latter part is profitable to read for an old man as well as for he man in his best years and for the young man.

The Sheikh, who gives good advice to the creatures of God the Great! He the sage, the savant, the first of the men of his time, speaks as follows on this subject; listen then to his words:

He who makes it a practice to eat every day fasting the yolks of eggs, without the white part, will find in this aliment an energetic stimulant towards coitus. The same is the case with the man who during three days eats of the same mixture with onions.

He who foils asparagus, and then fries them in fat, and then pours upon them the yolks of eggs with pounded condiments, and eats every day of this dish, will grow very strong for the coitus, and find in it a stimulant for his amorous desires.

He who peels onions, puts them into a saucepan, with the condiments and aromatic substances, and fries the mixture with oil and yolks of eggs, will acquire a surpassing and invaluable vigor for the coitus, if he will partake of this dish for several days.

Camel's milk mixed with honey and taken regularly develops a vigor for copulation which is unaccountable and causes the virile member to be on the alert night and day.

He who for several days makes his meals upon eggs boiled with myrrh, coarse cinnamon, and pepper, will find his vigor with respect to coition and erections greatly increased. He will have a feeling as though his member would never return to a state of repose.

A man who wishes to copulate during the whole night, and whose desire, having come on suddenly, will not allow him to prepare himself and follow the regimen just mentioned, may have recourse to the following recipe. He must get a great number of eggs, so that he may eat to surfeit, and fry them with fresh fat and butter; when done he immerses them in honey, working the whole mass well together. He must then eat of them as much as possible with a little bread, and he may be certain that for the whole night his member will not give him any rest.

On this subject, the following verses have been composed:

The member of Abou el Heiloukh has remained erect
For thirty days without a break, because he did eat onions.
Abou el Heidja has deflowered in one night
Once eighty virgins, and he did not eat or drink between,
Because he'd surfeited himself first with chick-peas,
And had drunk camel's milk with honey mixed.
Mimoun, the Negro, never ceased to spend his sperm while he
For fifty days without a truce the game was working.
How proud he was to finish such a task!
For ten days more he worked it, not was he yet surfeited,
But all this time he ate but yolk of eggs and bread.

The deeds of Abou el Heiloukh, Abou el Heidja and Mimoun, just cited, have been justly praised, and their history is truly marvelous. So I will make you acquainted with it, please God, and thus complete the signal services which this work is designed to render to humanity.

The History of Zohra

The Sheikh, the protector of religion (God, the Highest, be good to him!), records that there lived once in remote antiquity an illustrious King who had numerous armies and immense riches.

This King had seven daughters remarkable for their beauty and perfections. These seven had been born one after another, without any male infant between them.

The kings of the time wanted them in marriage, but they refused to be married. They wore men's clothing, rode on magnificent horses covered with gold-embroidered trappings, knew how to handle the sword and the spear, and bore men down in single combat. Each of them possessed a splendid palace with the servants and slaves necessary for such service, for the preparation of meat and drink, and other necessities of that kind.

Whenever a marriage offer for one of them was presented to the King, he never failed to consult with her about it; but they always answered, "That shall never be."

Different conclusions were drawn from these refusals, some in a good sense, some in a bad one.

For a long time no positive information could be gathered of the reasons for this conduct, and he daughters persevered in acting in the same manner until the death of their father. Then the oldest of them was called upon to succeed him, and

Positions for Intercourse

There is no doubt that the optimal positions for the most pleasurable acts of intercourse are the ones in which the couple's bodies touch as much as possible and enable each one to caress, nibble, kiss, suck and clasp the other. These positions must not only allow the man to insert his penis as deeply as possible into the woman's vagina, but also to ensure that its base rubs and presses on the clitoris the entire time. This is the best formula for couples to pleasure themselves and each other.

The most common position is when the woman lies on her back and the man lies on top of her in the same direction. She opens her legs to give him access to her vagina, and he lies between them. He has to support his weight on his knees and elbows, otherwise he will squash her – particularly if she is small. This position is liable to become uncomfortable for the man, however, especially if the lovemaking continues for a long time. To this end, the bed should be sufficiently soft, otherwise the man will end up with painful knees and elbows, which will detract from his pleasure.

received the oath of fidelity from all his subjects. This accession to the throne resounded through all the countries.

The name of the eldest sister was Fouzel Djemal (the flower of beauty); the second was called Soltana el Agmar (the queen of the moons); the third, Bediaat el Djemal (the incomparable in beauty); the fourth, Ouarda (the rose); the fifth, Mahmouda (the praiseworthy); the sixth Kamela (the perfect); and finally, the seventh, Zohra (the beauty).

Zohra, the youngest, was at the same time the most intelligent and judicious.

She was passionately fond of the chase, and one day as she was riding through the fields she met on her way a cavalier, who saluted her, and she returned his salute; she had some twenty men in her service with her. The cavalier thought it was the voice of a woman he had heard, but as Zohra's face was covered by a flap of haik, he was not certain, and said to himself, "I would like to know whether this is a woman or a man." He asked on of the princess's servants, who dissipated his doubts. Approaching Zohra, he then conversed pleasantly with her till they made a half for breakfast. He sat down near her to partake of the repast.

Disappointing the hopes of the cavalier, the princess did not uncover her face, and, pleading that she was fasting, ate nothing. He could not help admiring secretly her hand, the gracefulness of her waist, and the amorous expression of her eyes. His heart was seized with a violent love.

When the man wants to penetrate her vagina, the woman should raise her knees toward her breasts and hold her thighs as far apart as she can. When the man is inside her, she can lower her legs and wrap them around him, with her heels on his bottom. This will alleviate the tension in her spread thighs.

One of the drawbacks of this position is that the man, who is resting on his elbows, cannot use his arms freely to caress and fondle the woman. However, he can do so briefly with one hand at a time, touching her thighs, legs, armpits, belly and so on, which will respond to his caresses.

The advantage of this position is the proximity of the couple's bodies. They touch and rub each other constantly – and the movements of the man's chest on the woman's breasts will stimulate her nipples to be come erect and aroused. He should be aware of this and make deliberate side-to-side movements.

Kissing is also a cinch in this position – the couple can kiss as much and as deeply as they want, and this also enflames their passion. Furthermore, the man can often bend his head and nibble at one of the woman's breasts, which can set her off like a

The following conversation took place between them:

THE CAVALIER: Is your heart insensible for friendship?

ZOHRA: It is not proper for a man to feel friendship for a woman; for if their hearts once incline towards each other, libidinous desires will soon invade them, and with Satan enticing them to do wrong, their fall is soon known by everyone.

THE CAVALIER: It is not so, when the affection is true and their intercourse pure without infidelity or treachery.

ZOHRA: If a woman gives way to the affection she feels for a man, she becomes an object of slander for the whole world, and of general contempt, whence nothing arises but trouble and regrets.

THE CAVALIER: But our love will remain secret, and in this retired spot, which may serve us as our place of meeting, we shall have intercourse together unknown to all.

ZOHRA: That may not be. Besides, it could not so easily be done, we should soon be suspected, and the eyes of the whole world would be turned upon us.

THE CAVALIER: But love, love is the source of life. The happiness, that is, the meeting, the embraces, the caresses of lovers. The sacrifice of the fortune, and even of the life for your love.

ZOHRA: These words are impregnated with love, and your smile is seductive; but you would do better to refrain from similar conversation.

THE CAVALIER: Your word is emerald and your counsels

firecracker during orgasm. This is possible if the man doesn't have to bend his neck down too far.

During intercourse, it is the man's job to be in perpetual motion – with his entire body. His mouth is busy kissing, licking and sucking; his hands are roaming all over his partner's body, pleasuring her with his caresses and touches; his organ is thrusting at different speeds and at different depths to keep her titillated and stimulated and to help her along the path to her climax. It is imperative for the man to know how to prolong and intensify her ecstasy during orgasm.

After her orgasm, when the woman is in a state of exhaustion and often immobility, it is up to the man to continue thrusting gently inside her, as well as kissing and fondling her. This will help her recover from her exhaustion. Now is the time for him to display particular tenderness to her – by whispering sweet nothings and kissing her gently. She will respond to his consideration and affection, and soon the flames of her passion will be rekindled.

In the case of a thin, delicate woman, the man

are sincere. But love has now taken root in my heart, and no one is able to tear it out. If you drive me from you I shall assuredly die.

ZOHRA: For all that you must return to your place and I to mine. If it pleases God we shall meet again.

Then they separated, bidding each other adieu, and returned each of them to their dwelling.

The cavalier's name was Abou el Heidja. His father, Kheiroun, was a great merchant and immensely rich, whose habitation stood isolated beyond the estate of the princess, a day's journey distant from her castle. About el Heidja returned home, could not rest, and put on again his temeur when the night fell, took a black turban, and buckled his sword on under his temeur. Then he mounted his horse, and, accompanied by his favorite Negro, Mimoun, he rode away secretly under the cover of night.

They traveled all night without stopping until, on the approach of daylight, the dawn came upon them in sight of Zohra's castle. They then made a half among the hills, and entered with their horses into a cavern which they found there.

Abou el Heidja left eh Negro in charge of the horses and went in the direction of the castle, in order to examine its approaches; he found it surrounded by a very high wall. Not being able to get into it, he returned to some distance to watch those who came out. But the whole day passed away and he saw no one come out.

should remove his organ from her body, lie beside her and stroke her gently in order to help her recover. She will soon express her desire to resume the lovemaking.

There are a lot of women who don't want any breaks or rests between orgasms. They want the man to stay just where he is and keep on doing what he's doing. They seem to maintain a level of stimulation between orgasms as well. This can go on as long as the woman can endure and as long as the man can refrain from ejaculating.

A woman who knows the secrets of lovemaking also knows how to use her hands, fingers and mouth to prolong and intensify her man's pleasure when he finally reaches his own climax.

The Fountains of Pleasure

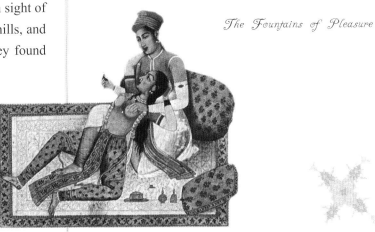

After sunset he sat himself down at the entrance of the cavern and kept on the watch until midnight; then sleep overcame him.

He was lying asleep with his head on Mimoun's knee, when the latter suddenly awakened him. "What is it?" he asked. "O my master," said Mimoun, "I have heard some noise in the cavern. Having ordered the Negro to wait for him while he was going to find out where it proceeded from, he took his saber and penetrated deeper into the cavern. He discovered a subterranean vault, into which he descended.

The road to it was nearly impracticable, on account of the stones which encumbered it. He contrived, however, after much trouble to reach a kind of crevice through which the light shone which he had perceived. Looking through it, he saw the Princess Zohra, surrounded by about a hundred virgins. They were in a magnificent palace dug out in the heart of the mountain, splendidly furnished and resplendent with godl everywhere. The maidens wee eating and drinking and enjoying the pleasures of the table.

Abou el Heidja said to himself, "Alas! I have no companion to assist me at this difficult moment." Under the influence of this reflection, he returned to his servant, Mimoun, and said to him, "Go to my brother before God, Abou el Heiloukh, and tell him to come here to me as quickly as he can." The servant forthwith mounted upon his horse, and rode through the remainder of the night.

> How many a lover with his eyebrows speaketh
> To his beloved, as his passion pleadeth:
> With flashing eyne [eyes] his passion he inspireth
> And well she seeth [sees] what his pleading needeth.
> How sweet the look when each on other gazeth;
> And with that swiftness and how sure it speedeth:
> And this with eyebrows all his passions writeth;
> And that with eyeballs all his passion readeth.
>
> *The Arabian Nights*

Of all his friends, Abou el Heiloukh was the one whom Abou el Heidja liked best; he was the son of the Vizir. This young man and Abou el Heidja and the Negro, Mimoun, passed as the thee strongest and most fearless men of their time, and no one ever succeeded in overcoming them in combat.

When the Negro Mimoun came to his master's friend, and had told him what happened, the latter said, "Certainly, we belong to God and shall return to him." Then he took his saber, mounted his horse, and taking his favorite Negro with him, he made his way, with Mimoun, to the cavern.

Aboul el Heidja came out to meet him and bed him welcome, and having informed him of the love he bore to Zohra, he told him of his resolution to penetrate forcibly into the palace, of the circumstances under which he had taken refuge in the cavern, and the marvelous scene he had witnessed while there. Abou el Heiloukh was dumb with surprise.

At nightfall they heard singing, boisterous laughter, and animated talking. Abou el Heidja said to his friend, "Go to the end of the subterranean passage and look. You will then make excuse for the love your brother." Abou el Heiloukh, stealing softly down to the lower end of the grotto, looked into the interior of the palac, and was enchanted with the sight of these virgins and their charms. "O brother," he asked, "which among these women is Zohra?"

Abou el Heidja answered, "The one with the irreproachable shape, whose smile is irresistible, whose cheeks are roses, and whose forehead is resplendently white, whose head is encircled by a crown of pearls, and whose garments sparkle with gold. She is seated on a throne encrusted with rare stones and nails of silver , and she is leaning her head upon her hand."

"I have observed her of all the others," said Abou el Heiloukh, as though she were a standard or a blazing torch. "But, O my brother, let me draw your attention to a matter which appears not to have struck you." "What is it?" asked Abou el Heidja. His friend replied, "It is very certain, O my brother, that licentiousness reigns in this palace. Observe that these people come here only at night-time, and that this is a retired place. There is every reason to believe that it is exclusively consecrated to feasting, drinking and debauchery, and if it was your idea that you could have come to her you love by any other way than the one on which we are now, you would have found that you had deceived yourself, even if you had found means to communicate with her by the help of other people." "And why so?" asked Abou el Heidja. "Because," said his friend, "as far as I can see, Zohra solicits the affection of young girls, which is proof that she can have no inclination for men, nor be responsive to their love."

O Abou el Heiloukh," said Abou el Heidja, "I know the value of your judgment, and it is for that I have sent for you., You know that I have never hesitated to follow your advice and counsel!" O my brother," said the son of the Vizir, "if

God had not guided you to this entrance of the palace, you would never have been able to approach Zohra. But from here, please God! We can find our way."

Next morning, at sunrise, they ordered their servants to make a breach in that place, and managed to get everything out of the way that could obstruct the passage. This done they hid their horses in another cavern, safe from wild beasts and thieves; then all the four, the two masters and the two servants, entered the cavern and penetrated into the palace, each of them armed with saber and buckler. They then closed up again the breach, and restored its former appearance.

Now they found themselves in darkness, but Abou el Heiloukh, having struck a match, lighted one of the candles, and they began to explore the palace in every sense. It seemed to them the marvel of marvels. The furniture was magnificent. Everywhere there were beds and couches of all kinds, rich candelabra, splendid lusters, sumptuous carpets, and tables covered with dishes, fruits and beverages.

When they had admired all these treasures, they went on examining the chambers, counting them. There was a great number of them, and in the last one they found a secret door, very small, and of appearance which attracted their attention. Abou el Heiloukh said, "This is very probably the door which communicates with the palace. Come, O my brother, we will await the things that are to come in one of these chambers." They took their position in a cabinet difficult of access, high up, and from which one could see without being seen.

So they waited till night came on. At that moment the secret door opened, giving admission to a negroes carrying a torch, who set alight all the lusters and candelabra, arranged the beds, set the plates, placed all sorts of meats upon the tables, with cups and bottles, and perfumed the air with the sweetest scents.

Soon afterwards the maidens made their appearance. Their gait denoted at the same time indifference and languor. They seated themselves upon the divans, and the negress offered them meat and drink. They ate, drank, and sang melodiously.

Then the four men, seeing them giddy with win, came down from their hiding place with their sabers in their hands, brandishing them over the heads of the maidens. They had first taken care to veil their faces with the upper part of the haik.

"Who are these men," cried Zohra, "who are invading our dwelling under cover of the shades of the night? Have you risen out of the ground, or did you descend from the sky? What do you want?"

"Coition!" they answered.

"With whom?" asked Zohra.

"With you, O apple of my eye!" said Abou el Heidja, advancing.

Zohra: "Who are you?"

"I am Abou el Heidja."

Zohra: "But how is it you know me?"

"It is I who met you while out hunting at such and such a place."

Zohra: "But what brought you hither?"

"The will of God the Highest!"

At this answer Zohra was silent, and set herself to think of a means by which she could rid herself of these intruders.

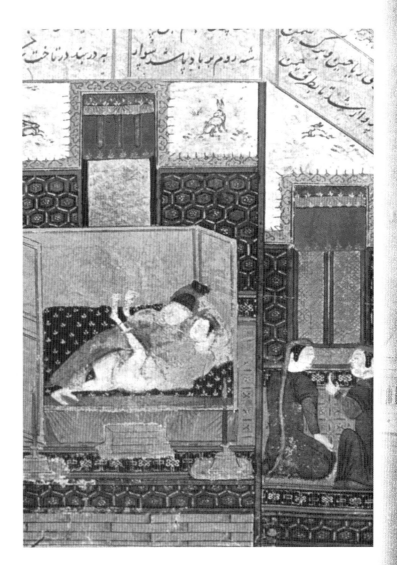

Now among the virgins that were present there were several whose vulvas were like iron barred, and whom no one had been able to deflower; there was also present a woman called Mouna (she who appeases the passion), who was insatiable as regards coition. Zohra thought to herself, "It is only by a stratagem I can get fid of these men. By means of these women I will set them tasks which they will be unable to accomplish as conditions for my consent." Then turning to Abou el Heidja, she said to him, "You will not get possession of me unless you fulfill the conditions which I shall impose upon you." The four cavaliers at once consented to this without knowing them, and she continued, "But, if you do not fulfill them, will you pledge your word that you will be my prisoners, and place yourselves entirely at my disposition?" "We pledge our words!" they answered.

She made them take their oath that they would be faithful to their word, and then, placing her hand in that of Abou el Haidja, she said to him, "As regards you, I impose upon you the task of deflowering eighty virgins without ejaculating. Such is my will!" He answered, "I accept."

She let him then enter a chamber where there were several kinds of beds, and sent to him the eighty virgins in succession. Abou el Haidja deflowered them all, and so ravished in a single night the maidenhood of eighty young girls without ejaculating the smallest drop of sperm. This extraordinary vigor filled Zohra with astonishment, and likewise all those who were present.

The princess turning then to the Negro Mimoun, asked, "And this one, what is his name?" They said, "Mimoun." "Your task shall be," said the princess, pointing to Mouna, "to do this woman's business without resting for fifty consecutive days; you need not ejaculate unless you like: but if the excess of fatigue forces you to stop, you will not have fulfilled your obligations." They all cried out at the hardness of such a task; but Mimoun protested, and said, "I accept the condition, and shall come out of it with honor!" The fact was that this Negro had an insatiable appetite for the coitus. Zohra told him to go with Mouna to her chamber, impressing upon the latter to let her know if the Negro should exhibit the slightest trace of fatigue.

"And you, what is your name?" she asked the friend of

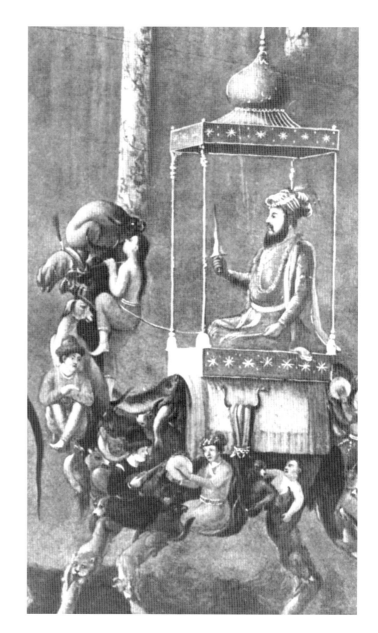

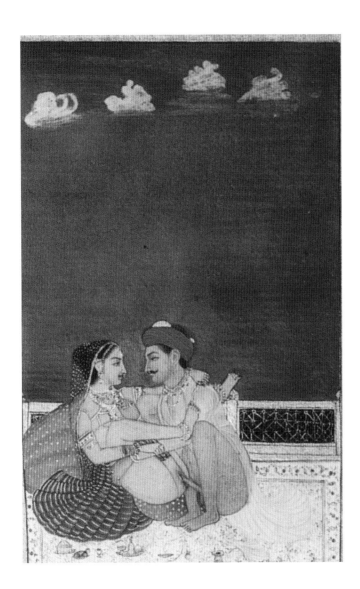

Abou el Heidja. "Abou el Heiloukh," he replied. "Well, then, Abou el Heiloukh, what I require of you is to remain here, in the presence of these women and virgins, for thirty consecutive days with your member during this period always in erection during day and night."

Then she said to the fourth, "What is your name?"

"Felah" (good fortune), was his answer. "Very well, Felah," she said, "you will remain at our disposition for any services which we may have to demand of you."

However, Zohra, in order to leave no motive for any excuse, and so that she might not be accused of bad faith, had asked them, first of all, what regimen they wished to follow during the period their trial. Aboul el Heidja had asked for only one drink – excepting water – camel's milk with honey, and, for nourishment, chick-peas cooked with meat and abundance of onions; and, by means of these aliments he did, by the permission of God, accomplish his remarkable exploit. Abou el Heiloukh demanded, for his nourishment, onions cooked with meat, and, for drink, the juice pressed out of pounded onions mixed with honey. Mimoun, on his part, asked fro yolks of eggs and bread.

However, Abou el Heidja claimed of Zohra the favor of copulating with her on the strength of the fact that he had fulfilled his engagement. She answered him, "Oh, impossible! The condition which you have fulled is inseparable from those which your companions have to comply with. The agreement must be carried out in its entirety, and you will find me true to my promise. But if one among you should fail in his task, you will all be my prisoners by the will of God!"

About el Jeidja gave way in the face of this firm resolve, and sat down among the girls and women, and ate and drank with the, while waiting for the conclusion of the tasks of his companions.

At first Zohra, feeling convinced that they would soon all be at her mercy, was all amiability and smiles. But when the twentieth day had come she began to show signs of distress; and on the thirteenth she could no longer restrain her tears. For on that day Abou el Heiloukh had finished his task, and, having come out of it honorably, he took his seat by the side of his friend among the company, who continued to eat tranquilly and to drink abundantly.

From that time the princess, who had now no other hope than in the failure of the Negro Mimoun, relied upon his becoming fatigued before he finished his work, She sent every day to Mouna for information, who sent word that the negro's vigor was constantly increasing, and she began to despair, seeing already Abou el Heidja and Abou el Heiloukh coming off as victors in their enterprises. One day she said to the two friends, "I have made inquiries about the Negro, and Mouna has let me know that he is exhausted with fatigue." At these words About el Heidja cried, "In the name of God! If he does not carry out his taste, aye, and if he does not go beyond it for ten days longer, he shall die the vilest of deaths!"

But his zealous servant never during the period of fifty days took any rest in his work of copulation, and kept going on, besides, for ten days longer, as ordered by his master. Mouna, on her part, had the greatest satisfaction as this feat had at last appeased her ardor for coition. Mimoun, having remained victor, could then take his seat with his companions.

Then said Abou el Heidja to Zohra, "See, we have fulfilled all the conditions you have imposed upon us. It is now for you to accord me the favors which, according to our agreement, were to be the price if we succeeded." "It is but too true!" answered the princess, and she gave herself up to him, and he found her excelling the most excellent.

As to the Negro, Mimoun, he married Mouna. Abou el Heiloukh chose, among all the virgins, the one whom he had found the most attractive.

They all remained in the palace, giving themselves up to good cheer and all possible pleasure, until death put an end to their happy existence and dissolved their union. God be merciful to them as well as to all Mussulmans! Amen!

It is to this story that the verses cited previously make allusion. I have given it here, because it testifies to the efficacy of the dishes and remedies, the use of which I have recommended, for giving vigor for coition, and all learned men agree in the acknowledging their salutary effects.

There are still other beverages of excellent virtue. I will describe the following: Take one part of the juice pressed out of pounded onions, and mix it with two parts of purified honey. Heat the mixture over a fire until the onion juice has disappeared and the honey only remains. Then take the residue from the fire, let it get cool, and preserve it for use when wanted. Then mix of the same one aoukia with three aouak of water, and let chick-pease be macerated in this fluid for one day and one night.

This beverage is to be partaken of during the winter and on going to bed. Only a small quantity is to be taken, and only for one day. The member of him who has drunk of it will not give him much rest during the night that follows. As to the man who partakes of it for several consecutive days, he will constantly have his member rigid and upright without intermission. A man with an ardent temperament out not to make use of it, as it may give him a fever. Nor should the medicine be used three days in succession except by old or cold-tempered men. And lastly, it should not be resorted to in summer.

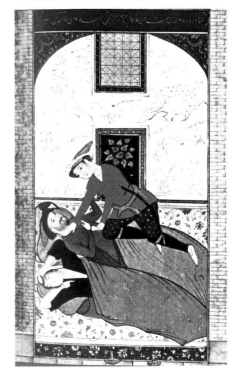

I certainly did wrong to put this book together;
But you will pardon me, nor let me pray in vain,
O God! Award no punishment for this on judgment day!
And thus, oh reader, hear me conjure thee to say: So be it!

The Perfumed Garden of the Sheikh Nefzaoui

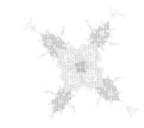

The Lustful Turk

'By this time I had recovered somewhat from my confusion, observing which the Dey, rising from the couch, said, in a low, determined tone, "How now, audacious slave, do you presume to oppose the will of thy master? Show again the least opposition to my desires and in an instant I shall have thee scourged properly for thy presumption. So mark me, slave!" After this menace he again seated himself and drew me upon his knees, with his arms round my waist. His determined manner of treating me had such an effect that I dared not resist his forcing his hand again into my breasts; but after he had sufficiently satisfied himself with feeling and moulding them, he suddenly turned his hands under my petticoats. His threats were now forgotten; I again strenuously resisted and struggled, whereupon he immediately desisted, and getting off the couch, with a small whistle which hung on his belt, he called in his black eunuchs, to one of whom he gave some orders in the Turkish language; the fellow went out, but quickly returned with a whip, which had about a dozen tails. I was now seized by the two eunuchs, who forced me across the couch with my face downwards; each of the eunuchs held me over the couch by the arm, so that I could not possibly get away. Having me thus secure and unmindful of my tears of entreaties, the Dey lifted up my clothes, and threw them all over my shoulders, leaving everything below my waist as naked as when I was born. Would you believe it, madame, he began to flog me in so unmerciful a manner that I could not retain my screams, of which he took not the least notice until he thought he had sufficiently punished my first offence. He then left off, and demanded if I would dare to oppose his wishes again. I could not at the moment have answered him, even if death had been the consequence. However, he allowed me very little time, but recommenced his flogging again, saying, "Oh, you are sullen are you? but I shall soon subdue you." Indeed, so painfully did I feel his lashes that at last I was able to cry that I would be submissive to his desires.

'I was directly relieved from the position I was in, and the eunuchs were dismissed, when the Dey, just as if nothing had happened, placed himself by my side; but, seeing I sat extremely uneasily from the soreness of the part he had so unmercifully whipped, he caused me to lie down on my side, laying himself beside me. He then drew me to his bosom and after kissing away my tears, sucking my lips and forcing his tongue into my mouth (which created great disgust in me), presently demanded if I was not married. I shuddered out an affirmative. "Curses on the Christian dog, I say, that has plucked your virginity!" he replied; "By Ali, I would have possessed it." You may be sure, madame, this made me blush, which made him remark how much my blushes increased my beauty. Again my lips became his prey. "How long have you been joined to the Christian dog?" demanded he, withdrawing his lips to let me answer him. I stammered out, "Only a month." "A month have thy blushes, then, been polluted. Well, I must be content with you as you are. Indeed, you are a feast fit for a monarch. How languishingly delicious is the modest cast of your eyes! Kiss me, trembler!" I dared not disobey, and, covered with blushes, joined my lips to his. He seemed much pleased with my obedience, and continued for some time most passionately kissing me. Whilst thus occupied, he slipped his right hand again under my petticoats and shift. A dreadful trembling seized me, but my fears prevented the least resistance, whilst his burning hand travelled over my most secret charms. Here was a change, madame, from the respect of poor Ludovico! The smallest favour was not granted to him until after the most urgent persuasions, whilst the Dey took every liberty he thought fit, and I believe thought he was conferring an honour upon me. He had now got his hand between my thighs and, drawing my lips closer to his, he desired me to open them a little wider, that he might have full command of the shrine of

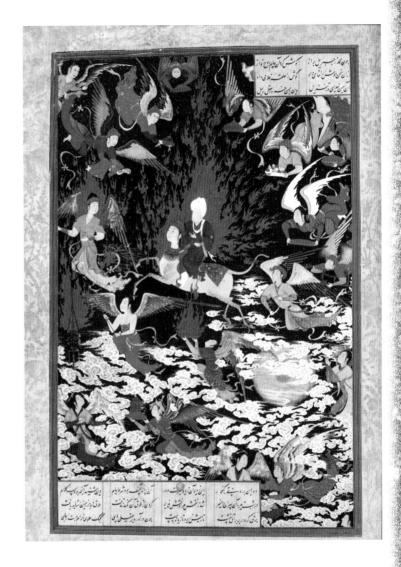

pleasure where he said he meant presently to sacrifice. I did not at the moment obey him. "How now," he cried, changing his tone from the soliciting to the commanding, "darest thou neglect my orders?" Oh, madame, the gradual extension of my thighs plainly spoke my fears. My tears flowed in torrents; my breasts heaved in convulsive agony. For a moment or so the Dey played with the soft down that crowns the mount of pleasure, and then slipped his finger between the lips of

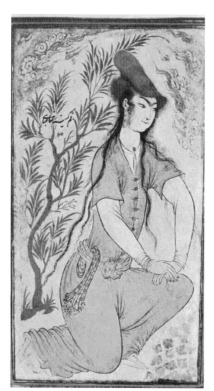

the road which until then had never been travelled, little dreaming of the discovery he was about to make. Indeed, on forcing his finger as far as he could into me, with great astonishment he found some difficulty in effecting entry, his efforts making me cry out that he hurt me. Surprised at my cries, he instantly started up, and forcing me on my back, extended my thighs to their utmost width, "Why, by Mahomet, you are a maid!" he cried, as he minutely examined me. "What punishment do you think you deserve for thus deceiving me as to your virginity?" Trembling and panting with shame and fear, I replied that I had not deceived him, as he had only asked how long I had been married, and I had told him the truth. "Then how is it," he demanded, "that your husband has not reaped his rights?" I at last confessed my maiden bashfulness had been the reason. At this the Dey laughed heartily, saying, "Whatever is the cause, holy Mahomet, I thank you for this unexpected treasure, but it shall not hang long on the stock [branch] for want of plucking." He then got off the couch, also assisting me to rise off my back; then applying the whistle to his mouth he summoned the same eunuchs, to whom he gave some directions as before. In obedience to his instructions they conducted me into a small room, every side of which was covered with glass: even the door at which I entered I could not discover when shut. In the centre of the room was a low dark-cushioned velvet couch, with one large cushion at the head; it was nothing but a plain broad couch, in the centre of which was fastened, properly extended, a beautiful white damask cloth.

'I was stripped in an instant by the eunuchs of every particle of my dress; they even untied the fillets [bands] which fastened up my hair; then, having reduced me to a complete state of nature, they retired, taking away my clothes. So much were my feelings overcome, that I was obliged to seat myself on the couch, or else I must have fallen. I was not doomed to wait long in suspense, for in a few seconds the Dey entered, as naked as myself. You, madame, no doubt well know how little ceremony, in cases of this kind, he uses. He took me in his arms, after kissing me, and told me he was now come to redress the wrongs I had suffered in the cruel neglect of my husband. "But," he said, "it will soon be repaired; you quickly shall taste such joys as your beauties so well deserve you should partake of. But why these tears and sighs? Is this the way you meet my caresses and kindness? Is this the return you make my generosity in preparing to teach you those pleasures which your husband has neglected. Come, come, let me have no more of this folly!" So drawing me to his bosom, he gently forced me on my back. "There now," he said, "lie down – no, not that way," seeing I was placing myself on my side, "it is on your back you must receive your first instructions. There, that's right; now open your soft thighs!" In an instant he was between them. I found I could not dare disobey. Finding my thighs were not quite extended enough, he soon widened them to his wish. I need not tell you how tremendously large the Dey is; turn in which way I would I could not help seeing in the glass the terrible pillar with which he was preparing to skewer me; quickly discovering the cause of my excessive alarm, whilst he was fixing its head between the lips of my virgin sheath, he tried by every kind of endearment to soothe me, assuring me the pain would be nothing – that my fears were unfounded; besides it was a sacrifice which nature had decreed, and once over the sweetest joys would be my reward; then why these foolish fears?

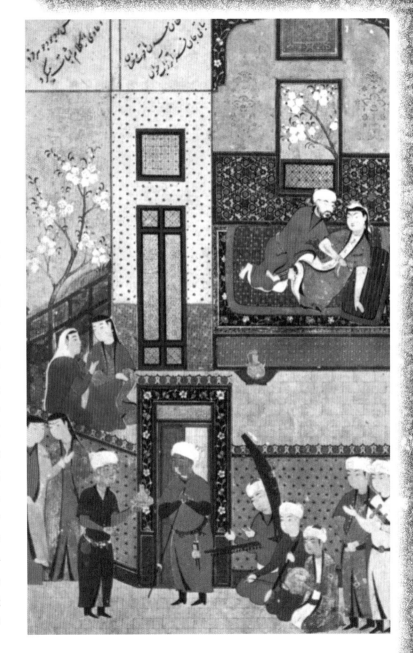

Thus did he soften me to his desires. The head of his instrument was no sooner fixed in the opening than by four or five sudden shoves he contrived to insert the whole of it entirely, so that I could not see any part of it as my face turned towards the glass. At this moment, his penetration was not deep enough to make me experience any great pain, but he, well knowing what was coming, forcibly secured one of his arms around my body.

'Everything was now prepared and favourable. My legs were glued to his, and I lay in his arms as it were insensible from despair, shame and confusion. He now began to improve his advantage by forcibly deepening his penetration; his prodigious stiffness and size gave me such dreadful anguish, from the separation of the sides of the soft passage by such a hard substance, that I could not refrain from screaming. Delicate as I was, he found great difficulty; but his Herculean strength in the end broke down all my virgin defences. My piercing cries spoke of my sufferings. In my agony I strove to escape, but the Dey, perfectly used to such attempts, easily foiled them by his able thrusts, and quickly buried his tremendous instrument too far within me to leave me any chance of escape. He now paid no kind of attention to my sufferings, but followed up his movements with fury, until the tender texture altogether gave way to his fierce tearing and rending, and one merciless, violent thrust broke in and carried all before it, sending his weapon, imbued and reeking with the

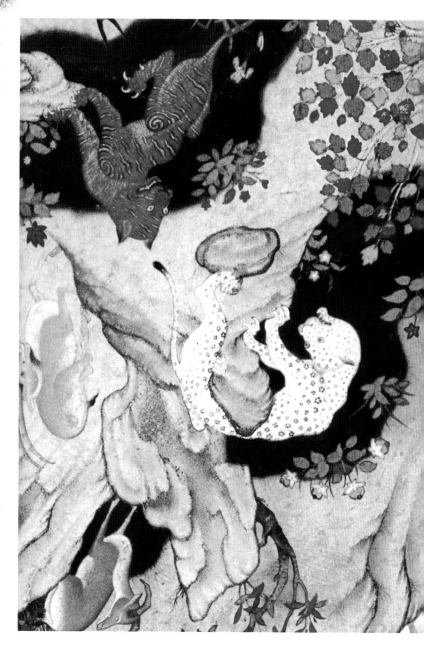

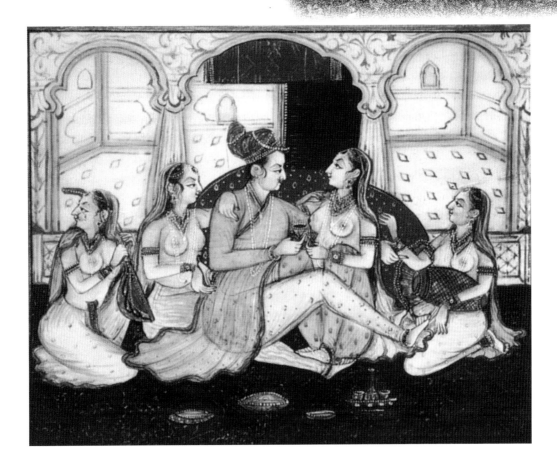

blood of my virginity, up to its utmost length in my body. The piercing shriek I gave proclaimed that I felt it up to the very quick; in short, his victory was complete.

'What my sufferings at first were I need not dwell upon, as no doubt you must have experienced them as painfully as myself, from his extraordinary size. It was also increased from the want of delicacy he used in subduing me. But my suffering did not seem to be any consideration with him, for he gave me no respite in his proceedings, but by enjoyment after enjoyment very soon blunted the sharpness of the pain, and ere [before] he withdrew from me I had sustained four assaults, which from their amorous fury had so stretched and opened me as to ensure I need never again complain on the score of suffering. Being satisfied on this point, he withdrew his shaft, and laying himself for a short time by my side, covered every part of me with burning kisses and caresses, assuring me that my sufferings were ended, and that I should shortly enjoy the pleasure of unmixed and pure delight in a manner that would reward me for all the anguish I had experienced in his fierce embraces. After reposing a short time on my bosom he got up and assisted me off the couch, which bore crimson evidence of my late loss. "Look," he cried, "my sweet slave," fondly pressing me in his arms, "I shall have your name worked in letters of gold on it, and it will then be deposited with a number of others that ornament a room in my harem. By virtue of this you are entitled to many privileges, which will be explained to you. Among others you are

forever exempt from any kind of attendance on my wives or chief sultanas, unless you choose to amuse yourself. But the slaves who will attend you will explain all the things which the blushing testimony of your chastity entitles you to." He then placed such a thrilling kiss on my lips that it threw me into the greatest confusion.

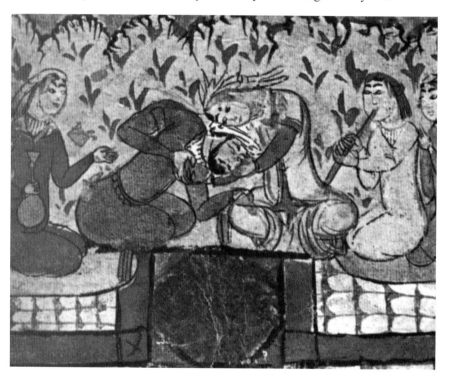

'He now called some Turkish slaves, who brought every kind of female clothing. They were not long in completing my toilet. This finished, he conducted me into a magnificent room, where refreshments were laid out. During the repast the Dey, by the most assiduous attention, strove to render himself agreeable, but as yet I could scarcely venture to look on him. It was still early in the morning. When we had finished our repast, he tenderly

enquired if I felt inclined to refresh myself by taking some repose alone. He could not have proposed anything more agreeable, which must have been evident by the immediate assent I gave to his offer. I was directly supported by him to a sleeping apartment, where, after again and again tenderly kissing me, he left me with a female slave, who soon undressed me; and in a soft slumber, which I soon fell into, my misfortunes were forgotten. My sleep was long and of course refreshing. I was awoken by the slave, who informed me that dinner was nearly ready; I got up and was assisted by her to dress. I then took dinner. After dinner the slave drew my attention to a large quantity of books, in my own language, which the Dey had caused to be sent to me. I found them to consist of our choicest authors. In my sitting-room he had occasioned a grand pianoforte to be placed, also an excellent lute, with a quantity of music, that I might not want amusement. I soon found several large portfolios of all kinds of prints, which alone were an inexhaustible store of amusement. The time imperceptibly passed in inspecting the various things which were placed for my recreation, until the slave reminded me that it was time I retired, as it was the Dey's intention to pass the night with me. What could I do?

Resistance was now out of the question; my virtue and modesty had received their mortal wounds. I had, even if I wished, no resource; indeed, nothing was left to me but to submit to my fate. Scarcely knowing where I was going, I was conducted to the bed-chamber, and soon was reduced to a proper state to meet the Dey's desires, being placed in bed in a state of panting, blushing confusion, very little different from that state I was in in the morning, when he debauched me. I was not long kept in suspense. I soon found myself in his strong arms. But, oh, how changed I now found him! All the authority of a master which he had so strongly assumed in the morning was not lost in the most passionate and tender regards of a most devoted and even submissive lover – even poor Ludovico could not be more so. I soon found his present proceedings more fatal to my morality than all the favours he had ravished from me by force under the influence of punishment. Indeed, I cannot explain the feeling he soon

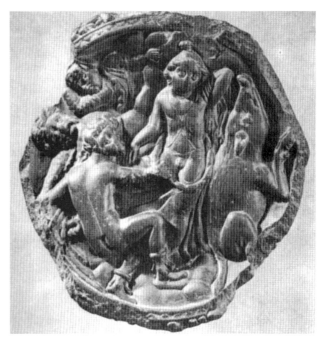

created. As I lay on his bosom he kissed me in a manner quite new, keeping my mouth to his several minutes, every now and then thrusting in his tongue and sucking mine. All the time he was doing this his hand was travelling over every part of my body with burning touches, creating the greatest disorder. The unopposed enjoyment of my lips, and feeling every secret beauty I possessed had now so heated his spirits, that to prevent the fluid that was boiling within him being improperly lost, it was absolutely necessary there should be no delay in my resigning to him the possession of the gates of pleasure. So far had his pressures and touches heated and inflamed me, that he found no obstacle in turning me on my back and again placing himself between my extended thighs. I scarcely recollect how it was, but I certainly felt at the moment he was fixing his instrument the soft prelude of pleasure illuminating within me. From trembling and fear I already began to desire; and, good God! how can I describe the surprise I felt when with one energetic shove he lodged himself up to the hilt in me without the smallest sensation of pain. Never, oh never shall I forget the delicious transports that followed the stiff insertion; and then, ah me! by what thrilling degrees did he, by his luxurious movements, fiery kisses, and strange touches of his hand in the most private parts of my body, reduce me to a voluptuous state of insensibility. I blush to say so powerfully did his ravishing instrument stir up nature within me, that by mere instinct I returned him kiss for kiss, responsively meeting his fierce thrusts, until the fury of the pleasure and ravishment became so overpowering that, unable longer to support the excitement I so luxuriously felt, I fainted in his arms with pleasure, Ludovico, the flogging, and everything else was entirely driven out of my head. So lively, so repeated were the enjoyments that the Dey caused me to participate in with him, I wondered how nature could have slumbered so long within me. I was lost in

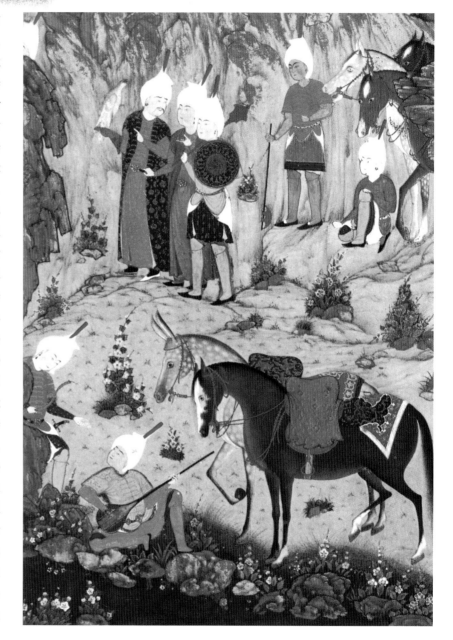

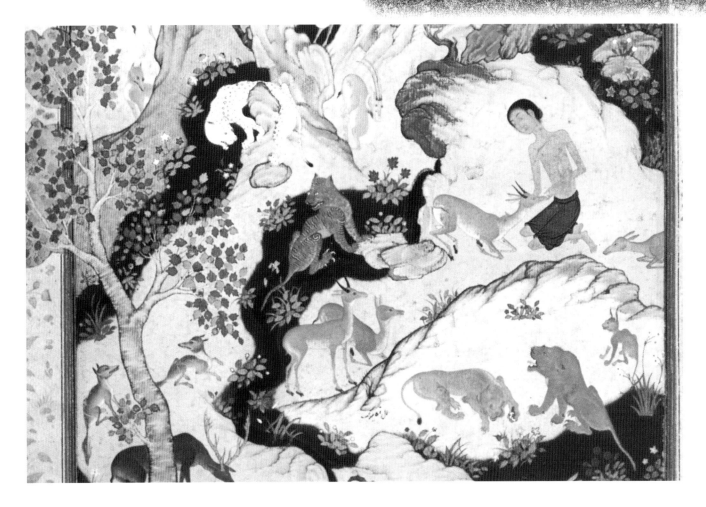

astonishment that in all the caresses I received from Ludovico he had not contrived to give the slightest alarm or feeling to nature. I could not help smiling at my ignorance when I considered the ridiculous airs I had assumed to Ludovico about my chastity. The Dey, indeed, had soon discovered my folly, and like a man of sense, took the proper method to subdue me. In this way, in one short night, you see, he put to the rout [banished] all my pure modest virgin scruples, rapturously teaching me the nature of love's sacred mysteries, and the great end for which we poor weak females are created. …''

The Lustful Turk

177

A Night in a Moorish Harem

Abdallah Pasha's Seraglio

Her British Majesty's ship Antler, of which I was in command, lay becalmed one afternoon off the coast of Morocco. I did not allow the steam to be raised for I knew the evening breeze would soon make toward the land.

Retiring to my cabin I threw myself upon the sofa. I could not sleep for my thoughts kept wandering back to the beautiful women of London and the favours which some of them had granted me when last on shore.

Months had elapsed since then and months more would elapse before I could again hope to quench, in the lap of beauty, the hot desire which now coursed through my veins and distended my genitals.

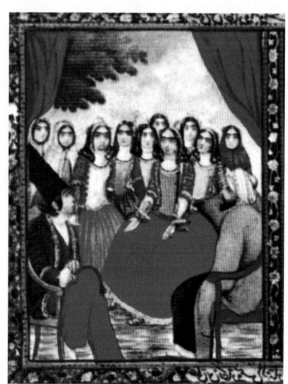

To divert my mind from thoughts at present so imperative I resolved to take a bath. Beneath the stern windows which lighted my cabin lay a boat, into which I got by sliding down a rope which held it to the ship. Then I undressed and plunged into the cool waves. After bathing I redressed, and reclining in the boat, fell asleep. When I awoke it was dark and I was floating along near the shore. The ship was miles away.

The rope which held the boat must have slipped when the breeze sprang up, and the people on the ship being busy getting underway had not noticed me. I had no oars and dared not use the sails for fear the Moorish vessels in sight would discover me. I drifted towards a large building which was the only one to be seen; it rose from the rocks near the water's edge. The approach to the place on which it stood seemed to be from the land side, and all the windows which I could see were high above the ground.

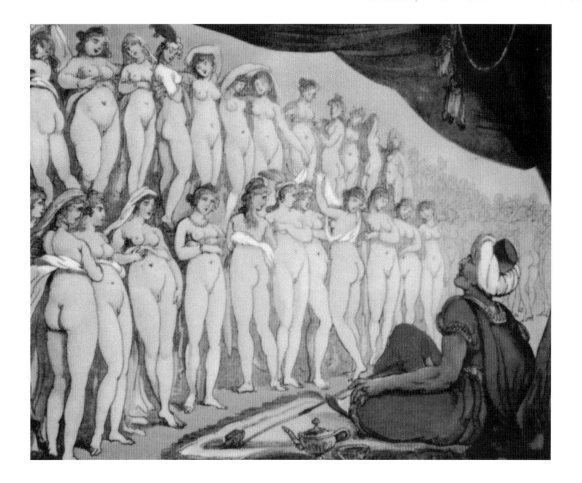

The keel of my boat soon grated on the sand and I hastened to pull it among the rocks for concealment, for it was quite possible I might be seized if discovered and sold into slavery. My plan was to wait for the land breeze just before dawn and escape to sea. At this moment I heard a whispered call from above. I looked up and saw two ladies looking down on me from the high windows above, and behind these two were gathered several others whom I could just see in the gloom.

'We have been watching you,' said the lady, ' and will try to assist you. Wait where you are.'

She spoke in French, which is the common medium of communication among the different nations inhabiting the

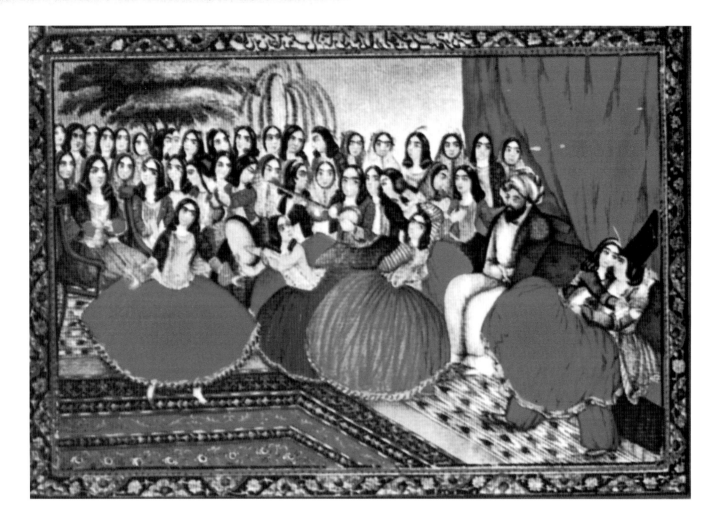

shores of the Mediterranean, and which had become familiar to me. I now thought this isolated building was a seraglio and I resolved to trust the ladies, who would run even more risk than myself in case of discovery.

After waiting some time, a rope of shawls was let down from the window and the same voice bid me climb. My discipline when a midshipman made this easy for me to do; I rose hand over hand and safely reached the window through which I was assisted by the ladies into the perfumed air of an elegant apartment richly furnished and elegantly lighted.

My first duty was to kiss the fair hands which had aided me, and then I explained the accident which had brought me among them and the plan I had formed for escape before dawn. I then gave my name and rank.

While doing this I had an opportunity to observe the ladies; there were nine of them and any one of them would have been remarked for her beauty. Each one of them differed from all the others in the style of her charms: some were large and some were small; some were slender and some plump, some blonde and some brunette, but all were bewitchingly beautiful. Each, too, was the most lovely type of a different nationality, for war and shipwrecks and piracy enable the Moorish Pashas to choose their darlings from under all the flags that float on the Mediterranean.

A lady whom they called Inez and whom, therefore, I took to be a Spaniard, answered me by bidding me in the name of all of them the warmest welcome.

'You are,' she said, ' in the seraglio of Abdallah, the Pasha of this district, who is not expected until tomorrow, and who will never be the wiser if his ladies seize so rare an opportunity to entertain a gentleman during his absence.' She added, 'We have no secrets or jealousy between ourselves,' smiling very significantly.

'That is very unusual,' said I. 'How can any of you know whether he has any secrets with the one he happens to be alone with?'

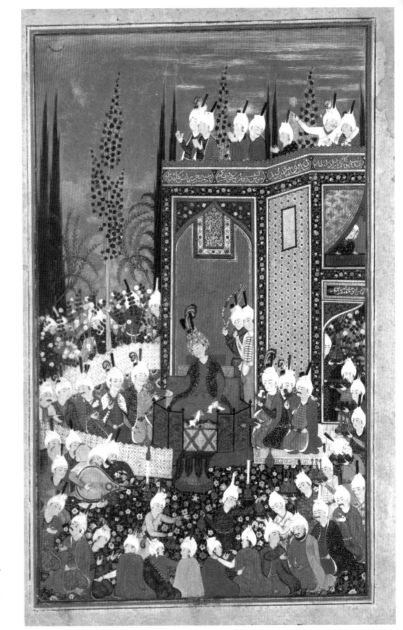

'But one of us is never alone with him,' said Inez. The blank look of consternation I had set them all laughing.

They were brimful of mischief and were evidently bent on making the most of the unexpected company of a young man. Inez put her hand on my sleeve. 'How wet you are,' said she. 'It will not be hospitable to allow you to keep on such wet clothes.'

My clothes were perfectly dry, but the winks and smiles that the young ladies exchanged as they began to disrobe me led me cheerfully to submit while they proceeded to divest me of every article of clothing.

When at length my shirt was suddenly jerked off they gave little affected screams and peeped thought their fingers at my shaft, which by this time was of most towering dimensions. I had snatched a hearty kiss from one and all of them as they had gathered round to undress me.

Inez now handed me a scarf which she had taken from her own fair shoulders. 'We can none of us bear to leave you,' she said, 'but you can only kiss one at a time; please throw this to the lady you prefer.'

Good heavens! Then it was true, that all of these beautiful women had been accustomed to be present when one of them was embraced.

'Ladies,' said I, 'you are unfair. You have

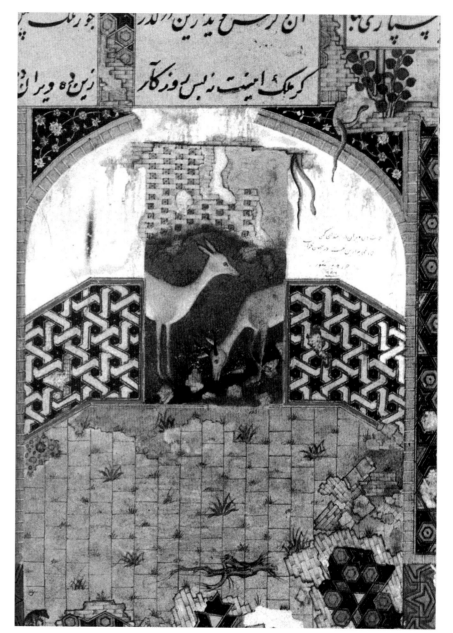

stripped me, but you keep those charms concealed which you offer to my preference. I am not sure now if you have any imperfections which you wish to keep covered.'

The ladies looked at one another, blushed a little, then nodded and laughed, then began undressing. Velvet vests, skirts of lawn and silken trousers were rapidly flung to the floor. Lastly, as if at a given signal, every dainty chemise was stripped off and some of the most lovely forms that ever floated though a sculptor's dream stood naked before me. Was I not myself dreaming, or had I in truth been suddenly transported amid the houses of the seventh heaven?

For a while I stood entranced, gazing at the charming spectacle. 'Ladies,' said I at last, 'it would be immodest in me to give preference when all are so ravishingly lovely. Please keep the scarf, fair Inez, and when I have paid a tribute to your fair charms, pass it yourself to another, till all have been gratified.'

'Did he say all?' cried a little brunette.

'All indeed!' cried the rest in chorus, bursting into laughter.

'Every one,' said I,' or I will perish in the attempt.'

Inez was standing directly in front of me; she was about nineteen, and of that rarest type

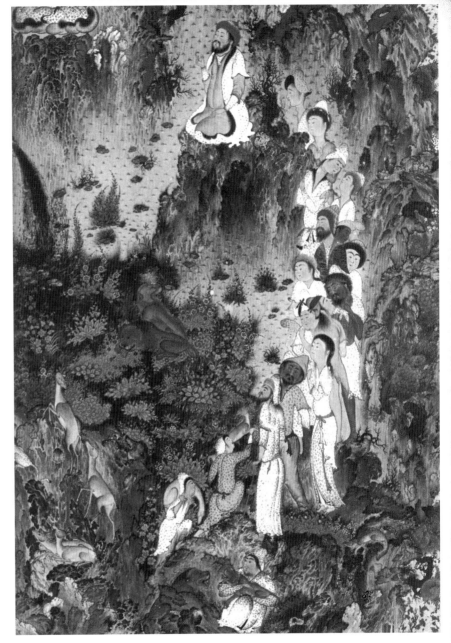

of Spanish beauty, partly derived from Flemish blood. Her eyes were sparkling brown, but her long hair was blonde. It was braided and coiled round the top of her head like a crown which added to her queenly appearance, for she was above the ordinary stature; her plump and well-rounded form harmonised with her height. Her complexion had the slight yellow tinge of rich cream, which was set off by the rosy nipples which tipped her full breasts and the still deeper rose of her lips and mouth.

She happened to be standing on one of the silken cushions which, singly and in piles, were scattered about the room in profusion. It made her height just equal to my own. As soon as I had made the speech last recorded, I advanced and folded her in my embrace.

Her soft arms were wound round me in response; and our lips met in a delicious and prolonged kiss, during which my shaft was imprisoned against her warm, smooth belly. Then she raised herself on tiptoe, which brought its crest amid the short, thick hair where the belly terminated. With one hand I guided my shaft to the entrance which welcomed it; with my other I held her plump buttocks toward me. Then she gradually settled on her feet again, and, as she did so, the entrance was slowly and delightfully effected in her moist, hot and swollen sheath. When she was finally on her feet again I could feel her throbbing womb resting on my shaft.

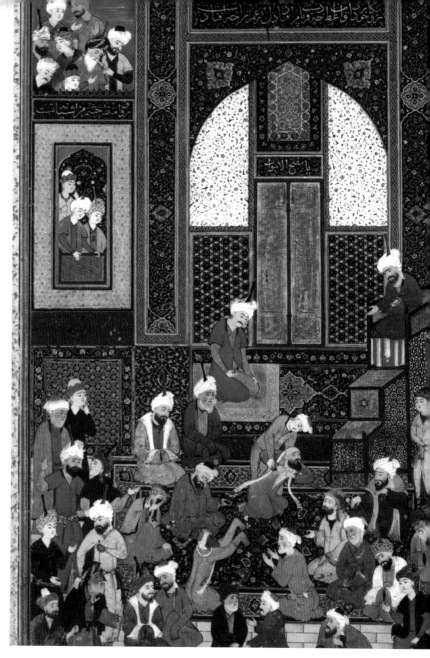

The other ladies had gathered round us; their kisses rained on my neck and shoulders, and the presence of their bosoms and bellies was against my back and sides – indeed they so completely sustained Inez and myself that I seemed about to mingle my being with them all at once. I had stirred the womb of Inez with but a few thrusts – when the rosy cheeks became a deeper dye, her eyes swam, her lips parted and I felt a delicious baptism of moisture on my shaft.

Then her head sank on my shoulder, the gathered sperm of months gushed from my crest so profusely that I seemed completely transferred with waves of rapture into the beautiful Spanish girl. Her sighs of pleasure were not only echoed by my own, but by those of all the ladies gathered around us in sympathy. They gently lowered us from this sustaining embrace to a pile of cushions. As they did so, with hardly any aid on our part, my diminished shaft was drawn out of Inez and, with it, some of my tributary sperm, which splashed on the floor.

'It was too bad of you, Inez, to take more than you can keep,' said one of the others. She said it in such a pitiful tone it convulsed us all with laughter. As for me, I now realised the rashness of the promise I had made them all, but they gaily joined hands round Inez and myself and began a circling dance, their round, white limbs and plump bosoms floating in the lamplight as they moved in cadence

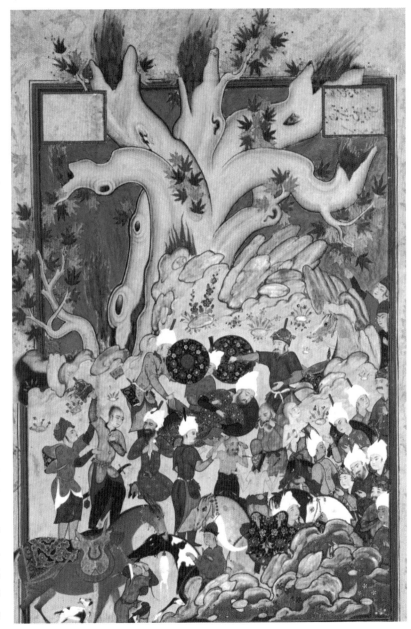

to a Moorish love song, in which they all joined. With my cheeks pillowed against the full breasts of Inez, I watched the charming circle, which was like a scene in fairy land. Bracelets and anklets of heavy fettered gold glittered on their arms and legs; rings, necklaces and earrings of diamonds and rubies, which they had in profusion, glistened at every movement.

Each one had her hair elaborately dressed in the style peculiarly becoming to herself and there were no envious garments to conceal a single charm. I urged them to prolong the bewitching spectacle again and again, which they obligingly did. Then they gathered around me, reclining to rest on the cushions as near as they could get, in attitudes which were picturesque and voluptuous.

When we were thus resting I frequently exchanged a kiss or caress with my fair companions, which I took care to do impartially. Then it occurred to me that I would like to hear from the lips of each the most interesting and voluptuous passage from their lives. Again these interesting ladies, after a little urging, consented, and Inez commenced.

A Night in a Moorish Harem

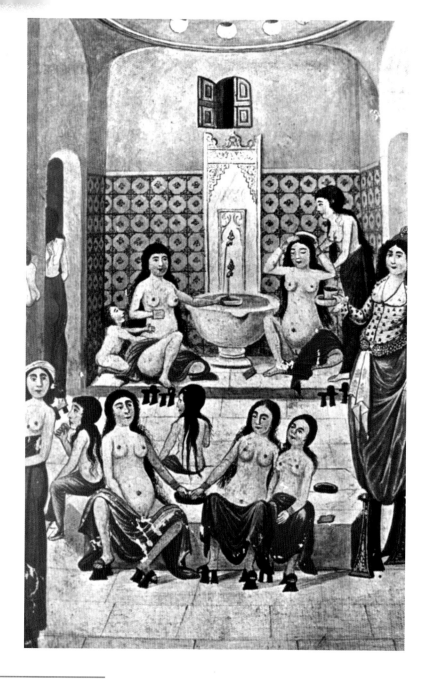

The Fountains of Pleasure

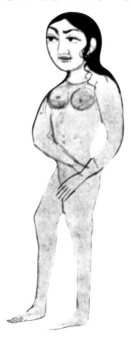

While tasting your sweetheart's saliva while kissing is delicious and stimulating, it can be revolting if you haven't rinsed your mouth. It's very important to do so directly after eating and before getting down to kissing. According to Muhammad, "the dirty mouths and bodies of men and women are liable to ruin their love." Moreover, Allah says that cleanliness is godliness.

What is good kissing? First, open your mouth wide and suck your partner's lips into it. Let your tongue go on a tour of her mouth, concentrating on the highly sensitive areas places between her lips and teeth. She should reciprocate, and while she is doing so, you should succumb to the sensations her tongue arouses in you. Don't rush. The secret of good intercourse is good kissing beforehand – it gets the woman in the right mood.

Joined mouths and synchronized breathing enhance your feeling for each other. Your shared breathing increases your passion, and you will be well on the way to the climax of your pleasure.

It's a very good idea to stroke your partner's perineum – that is, the region between the vulva and the anus – since this produces highly pleasurable sensations, especially during intercourse. In addition, while your penis is inside her vagina, you should insert your finger as well, since this creates more friction in the vagina and increases the pressure on the clitoris. This is an excellent technique for men with rather narrow penises or women with broad vaginas, or in cases of a position in which insufficient pressure is exerted on the clitoris.

In order to heighten the woman's pleasure, you should gently caress the very sensitive tissue of her anus. She may well experience pleasurable contractions there that will radiate to her vagina. Naturally, it is imperative that she wash her anus thoroughly before engaging in this activity.

The sensitive areas of the woman's inner thighs should not be neglected. As well as being very stimulating to look at, you should caress them with your hands, lips, tongue and teeth. You can do this while fondling her vagina in order to excite her. If you can pay attention to the woman's thighs during intercourse as well, it will increase her pleasure.

You should not stop at the woman's thighs: her calves and feet also beg for attention. Tickling and caressing her feet is a highly erotic stimulus.

Making your way northward from the woman's mons veneris, you will reach her waistline, which will also respond to your kisses and caresses. Turn her over and caress the region of her kidneys – she'll go wild with pleasure. While you are roaming from breasts to vagina, see that you pay suitable tribute to her belly and let your hands and mouth play there. Both of you will be stimulated and excited.

Armpits are a wonderful erogenous zone. Stroke and taste her there. When she is aroused, her armpits exude a particularly feminine odor that is reminiscent of that of her vagina. This will make you even more passionate.

Women love to have their backs rubbed and stroked. Have her lie on her stomach and then let your mouth and tongue make their way lightly up and down her spine, which is extremely sensitive. She'll go wild. Continue upward and bite her shoulders gently. It makes some women almost faint with pleasure.

One of the most exciting features of a woman's body is a beautiful neck. It's certainly an aphrodisiac for the male beholder. Try using your mouth on the back of her neck – especially if you're lying on top of her. Her ecstatic wriggling will be indescribably pleasurable for you, too.

Worship her face and all of its features with light kisses and caresses – whisper sweet nothings to her while doing so. Her ears are another wonderful erogenous zone. Don't flood them with saliva – just lick and nibble at them, and wait for the response.

Play with her hair by stroking it and pulling it gently while you bury your face in it. She will love the feeling, since her scalp is very sensitive.

Just like her inner thighs, you should not neglect the inner part of her upper arms. Caresses and kisses in that area will drive her wild, and make her hold on to you for dear life. Don't underestimate her palms and fingers: they are packed with nerve-endings and are a well-known erogenous zone.

The Fountains of Pleasure

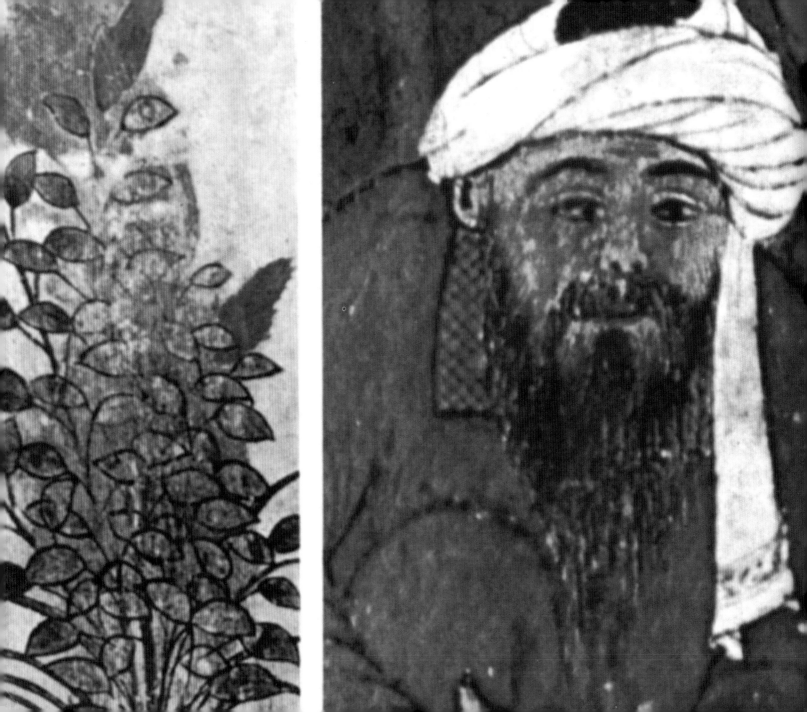

Contents

The Perfumed Garden of the Sheikh Nefzaoui   Translated by Sir Richard Burton

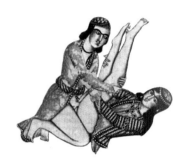

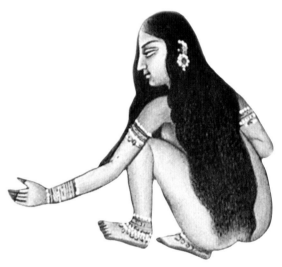

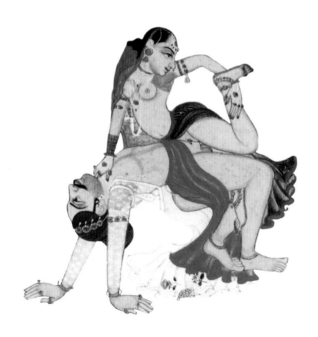